A Virtuous Life in Business

A Virtuous Life in Business

Stories of Courage and Integrity
in the Corporate World

Oliver F. Williams
and
John W. Houck
Editors

Rowman & Littlefield Publishers, Inc.

ROWMAN & LITTLEFIELD PUBLISHERS, INC.

Published in the United States of America
by Rowman & Littlefield Publishers, Inc.
4720 Boston Way, Lanham, Maryland 20706

British Cataloging in Publication Information Available

Library of Congress Cataloging-in-Publication Data

A Virtuous life in business / Oliver F. Williams and
    John W. Houck, editors.
        p.   cm.
    Papers from a symposium hosted by the Notre Dame Center
for Ethics and Religious Values in Business on April 2–3, 1990.
    1. Business ethics—Congresses.   2. Theological virtues—
Congresses.   3. Business—Religious aspects—Christianity—
Congresses.   I. Williams, Oliver F.   II. Houck, John W.
HF5387.V57   1992
174'.4—dc20   92–5513 CIP

ISBN 0–8476–7746–X (cloth : alk. paper)
ISBN 0–8476–7747–8 (pbk. : alk. paper)

Printed in the United States of America

 The paper used in this publication meets the minimum requirements of
American National Standard for Information Sciences—Permanence of
Paper for Printed Library Materials, ANSI Z39.48–1984.

To the many men and women
whose business stories of
virtue inspired this volume.

Contents

Preface

The Notre Dame Center for Ethics and Religious Values in Business hosted a symposium, *A Virtuous Life in the Business Story*, on April 2-3, 1990. Important scholars from a variety of disciplines discussed the recent trends in narrative theology and the theory of virtue, which may have much to contribute to the literature on the ethical dimension of business life.

The discussion in the ethics of business today is dominated by the two major theories of principle, the deontological and the utilitarian. Yet these theories may provide only a partial picture. The point here is that much of the behavior that is cited as exemplary in the corporate world, for example the Tylenol decisions by Johnson & Johnson or the Rely product recall decision by Procter and Gamble, is not sufficiently explained as just principled action. Rather, what made the top management of these firms corporate heroes in the eyes of many is that they exhibited uncommon virtue in maintaining allegiance to their principles. This was demonstrated, for example, in the *courage* to act to protect human welfare even in the midst of incomplete information, and in the *integrity* and *humility* in communicating with consumers about possible difficulties with a product.

The discussion of virtue often is given focus in narrative theology. In 1978 the Center published *Full Value: Cases in Christian Business Ethics* which brought narrative theology in dialogue with business practice. Now it is time to assess the contribution of narrative theology and theories of virtue on the current discussion of the ethics of management. Are the current attempts to develop the ethical focus of the managers of our private and public institutions adequate? Can a retrieval of a theory of virtue yield added clarity and insight to the literature? How is virtue best promoted in a corporate culture? These and other questions occupied the scholars and practitioners who authored the essays in this volume.

· · · · ·

The Center for Ethics and Religious Values in Business seeks to build bridges among business, business studies and the humanities. Its programs are designed to strengthen the Judeo-Christian ethical foundations in business and public policy decisions by fostering dialogue between academic and corporate leaders, and by research and publications. The Center is under the co-directorship of Oliver F. Williams, C.S.C. (theology), associate provost, and John W. Houck (business), professor of management, College of Business Administration.

In 1978, the Center published *Full Value: Cases in Christian Business Ethics,* which was the inaugural volume of Harper & Row's Experience and Reflection series. Michael Novak commented that the book "quite successfully juxtaposes the power of the Christian story, in its biblical immediacy, to concrete problems Christians in the world of business are likely to meet." James M. Gustafson wrote about *Full Value*: "Religious traditions provide, as these writers observe, a story, for example the Christian story, which informs our moral outlook, creates our moral vision, sustains our moral loyalties, and nurtures our moral character."

In 1980 the Center hosted a national symposium, *The Judeo-Christian Vision and the Modern Business Corporation.* The *Los Angeles Times* contrasted "the competitive success-oriented style necessary for corporate promotion with the traditional Christian view of the virtuous person." The *New York Times* reported that "there there would be no facile resolution to the conflict between the values of a just society and the sharply opposing values of successful corporations." Speakers at the symposium were:

John C. Bennett, Claremont School of Theology, and former president, Union Theological Seminary, New York; Catherine B. Cleary, director, AT&T, General Motors Corporation, Kraft Inc. and Northwestern Mutual Life Insurance, and former chair and chief executive officer, First Wisconsin Trust Company, Milwaukee; Richard Eells director, Center for the Study of the Corporation, Columbia University; Denis Goulet, O'Neill professor of education for justice, University of Notre Dame; James M. Gustafson, university professor, University of Chicago Divinity School; Kenneth P. Jameson, professor of economics, University of Notre Dame; Elmer Johnson, senior partner, Kirkland and Ellis, Chicago; Burton M. Leiser, professor of philosophy, Drake University; Enda McDonagh, Huisking professor in theological ethics, University of Notre Dame; Michael Novak, resident scholar, American Enterprise Institute, Washington, D.C.; James M. Schall, S.J., Department of Government, Georgetown University, and the Gregorian, Rome; S. Prakash Sethi, director, Center for Research in Business and Social Policy, University of Texas-Dallas; William P. Sexton, chair, Department of Management, University of Notre Dame; Edward R. Trubac, professor of finance and business economics, University of Notre Dame; Thomas Werge, chair, Department of English, University of Notre Dame; Charles Wilber, chair, Department of Economics, University of Notre Dame; and John Howard Yoder, professor of theology, University of Notre Dame.

A second symposium, *Co-creation: A Religious Vision of Corporate Power,* followed in 1982, focusing on Pope John Paul II's encyclical letter, *Laborem Exercens. Newsweek* characterized the conference as a "free marketplace of ideas" exploring a religious vision of corporate power. Contributors to this conference included:

Ernest J. Bartell, C.S.C., executive director, Helen Kellogg Institute for International Studies, University of Notre Dame; Thomas P. Carney, president, Metatech Corporation; John B. Caron, president, Caron International; Mary Cunningham, vice president, Joseph E. Seagram & Sons; Thomas R. Donahue, secretary-treasurer, AFL-CIO; Mark J. Fitzgerald, C.S.C., professor of economics, University of Notre Dame; Denis Goulet, O'Neill professor of education for justice, University of Notre Dame; Stanley Hauerwas, Department of Theology, University of Notre Dame; J. Bryan Hehir, director, Social Development and World Peace, U.S. Catholic Conference, Washington, D.C.; David Hollenbach, S.J., Weston School of Theology; Elmer W. Johnson, senior partner, Kirkland and Ellis, Chicago; Barry P. Keating, professor of finance and business economics, University of Notre Dame; Andrea Lea, I.H.M., dean, Continuing Education, Marygrove College, Detroit; George C. Lodge, Harvard Business School; Bernard Marchland, Department of Philosophy, Ohio Wesleyan University; Amata

I.H.M., financial vice president, I.H.M. Sisters of Monroe, Michigan; Michael Novak, resident scholar, American Enterprise Institute, Washington, D.C.; and Joseph A. Pichler, executive vice president, Dillon Companies, Inc.

In December 1983, the Center assisted the U.S. Bishops' Committee charged to write a pastoral letter on the economy by convening a three-day symposium, *Catholic Social Teaching and the American Economy.* The *Los Angeles Times* observed: "About one-third of the major speakers represented conservative viewpoints, the remainder voiced moderate-to-liberal positions." The *New York Times* reported that "contentiousness is commonplace here at Notre Dame....And when dozens of business leaders, theologians and academics lined up against each other at the university this week, the debate over the economy was fought as hard as any gridiron encounter." More than 250 people attended the meeting, including the five bishops who were to draft the letter. Joining in the drafting of the working papers, and providing a religious commentary and perspectives on the theme of the symposium, were:

Gar Alperovitz, co-director, National Center for Economic Alternatives; Ernest J. Bartell, C.S.C., executive director, Helen Kellogg Institute for International Studies, University of Notre Dame; C. Fred Bergsten, director, Institute for International Economics; Daniel Rush Finn, Department of Theology and Department of Economics and Business Administration, St. John's University, Collegeville, Minnesota; Joe Holland, co-director, Center for Concern; David Hollenbach, S.J., Weston School of Theology; Elmer W. Johnson, chief counsel and group executive-public affairs, General Motors Corporation; F. Ray Marshall, Lyndon B. Johnson School of Public Affairs, University of Texas at Austin; Dennis P. McCann, professor of religious studies, DePaul University; Michael Novak, resident scholar, American Enterprise Institute; Graciela Olivarez, attorney-at-law, Albuquerque, New Mexico; Rudy Oswald, research director, AFL-CIO; Peter G. Peterson, chair, Lehman Brothers Kuhn Loeb Inc.; Joseph A. Pichler, president, Dillon Corporation, Inc.; Marina von Neumann Whitman, vice president and chief economist, General Motors Corporation; and Oliver F. Williams, C.S.C., University of Notre Dame.

Catholic Social Teaching and the Common Good was the theme of a 1986 symposium to explore the possible retrieval of the notion of "the common good" in philosophical-economic discourse. Ralph McInerny saw the concept of the common good as needed "to draw attention to flaws in our economic thinking and policies as well as to make positive suggestions that will be manifestly in line with our tradition." *New Catholic World* wrote: "a collection of eighteen essays...by social scientists, theologians, philosophers, business faculty, and television producers. The essays represent different points of view from both theoretical and practical perspectives....It would be a valuable contribution to Catholic social teaching if all it did was to make people aware that a concept of the common good once was alive and well. It does much more than that." Contributors to the conference included:

Gar Alperovitz, co-director, National Center for Economic Alternatives; Ernest J. Bartell, C.S.C., executive director, Helen Kellogg Institute for International Studies, University of Notre Dame; Bette Jean Bullert, independent television producer; Gerald F. Cavanagh, S.J., Department of Management, University of Detroit; John J. Collins, professor of theology, University of Notre Dame; John W. Cooper, dean, Academic Affairs, Bridgewater College, Virginia; William J. Cunningham, research economist, AFL-CIO; Charles E. Curran, Department of Theological Ethics, Catholic University of America; Richard T. De George, university distinguished professor of philosophy, University of Kansas; Peter Mann, producer of television programs for the Diocese of Rockville Center, New York; Dennis P. McCann, professor of religious studies, DePaul University; Ralph McInerny, Grace professor of medieval studies, and director, Jacques Maritain Center, University of Notre Dame; Richard J. Neuhaus, director, The Center on Religion and Society, New York City; Michael Novak, resident scholar, American Enterprise Institute; David Vogel, Department of Business Administration, University of California-Berkeley; Charles C. West, Stephen Colwell professor of Christian ethics, Princeton Theological Seminary; Charles K. Wilber, professor of economics, University of Notre Dame; and J. Philip Wogaman, professor of Christian social ethics, Wesley Theological Seminary, Washington, D.C.

The 1987 symposium focused on *Ethics and the Investment Industry*. Much has been written in the eighties about the misdeeds of actors in the investment community; suggestions for legislative reform abound. Very little has been said about the ethical vision and institutional bonding that form the context for a humane capitalism. It is these themes, as well as the appropriate market and legal aspects, that were explored at Notre Dame. *America* said of *Ethics and the Investment Industry* that it "will be an important reference for future participants in the international business community." The speakers and panelists were:

G. Robert Blakey, O'Neill professor, University of Notre Dame School of Law; George P. Brockway, former chair, W.W. Norton and Company; Gerald F. Cavanagh, S.J., professor of management, University of Detroit; Richard T. De George, university distinguished professor of philosophy, University of Kansas; Edward J. Epstein, contributing editor, Manhattan, Inc.; Kirk O. Hanson, Stanford Graduate School of Business; Gregg Jarrell, former chief economist of the Securities and Exchange Commission; Burton M. Leiser, Edward J. Mortola professor of philosophy, Pace University; Dennis P. McCann, professor of religious studies, DePaul University; Patricia A. O'Hara, professor of law, University of Notre Dame School of Law; John J. Phelan, Jr., chair of the boards of the New York Stock Exchange and the New York Futures Exchange; Frank K. Reilly, Bernard J. Hank professor of business administration, University of Notre Dame; Donald W. Shriver, Jr., president, New York Union Theology Seminary; Paul E. Tierney, Jr., partner, Gollust, Tierney and Oliver; Alfred C. Morley, president and chief executive officer, The Institute of Chartered Financial Analysts, and president, Financial Analysts Federation; Clarence C. Walton, Charles Lamont Post distinguished professor of ethics and professions, American College, and former president, Catholic University; John G. Weithers, chair of the board, Midwest Stock Exchange; Robert Wilmouth, president and chief executive officer, National Futures Association, and chair, LaSalle National Bank, Chicago.

Described by one noted theologian as "the most powerful leader in the world," Pope John Paul II has authored two documents that may have much to say to our times: *On Human Work (Laborem Exercens)* and *On Social Concern (Sollicitudo Rei Socialis)*. Is the religious social teaching in these documents in such contrast to the prevailing wisdom of political economy that they might properly be called countercultural? Does this teaching offer a new vision, a strikingly different way of interpreting economic events? To address these issues, the Notre Dame Center for Ethics and Religious Values in Business convened a symposium in 1989 on the recent teaching of the Catholic Church on economic ethics. The assembled business executives, labor leaders and scholars included:

Ernest J. Bartell, C.S.C., executive director, Helen Kellogg Institute for International Studies, University of Notre Dame; Robert Benne, professor of philosophy and religion, Roanoke College, Virginia; Richard T. De George, professor of philosophy, University of Kansas; Teresa Ghilarducci, professor of economics, University of Notre Dame; Denis Goulet, O'Neill professor of education for justice, University of Notre Dame; Leslie Griffin, professor of theology, University of Notre Dame; J. Bryan Hehir, counselor for social policy, U.S. Catholic Conference, Washington, D.C.; John Langan, S.J., professor of Christian ethics, Woodstock Theological Center, Georgetown University; Dennis P. McCann, professor of religious studies, DePaul University; Michael Novak, senior scholar, American Enterprise Institute, Washington, D.C.; James E. Post, professor of management and public policy, Boston University; Ricardo Ramirez, C.S.B., bishop of Las Cruces, New Mexico; S.Prakash Sethi, professor of business policy, Baruch College, New York; Paul Steidlmeier, professor of management, State University of New York; Lee A. Tavis, C.R. Smith professor of finance, University of Notre Dame; Theodore R. Weber, professor of theology, Emory University; Preston Williams, professor of theology and contemporary change, Harvard Divinity School; J. Philip Wogaman, professor of Christian social ethics, Wesley Theological Seminary, Washington, D.C.; and John Howard Yoder, professor of theology, University of Notre Dame.

The University of Notre Dame and its Center for Ethics and Religious Values in Business hosted an international symposium in 1991 to anticipate the sesquicentennial celebration of the University (1842-1992) and to focus on another timely anniversary—one hundred years of Catholic Social Thought.

One writer suggested that Catholic Social Thought is the best thing the Catholic Church has done in the last one hundred years! Although disputed and controversial, this observation by our commentator clearly pointed to the importance of Catholic Social Thought as a powerful voice of social assessment and leadership. The tradition of the Church speaking out to the world on social justice questions started in 1891 with Leo XIII's *Rerum Novarum*; there was the U.S. Bishops' 1919 statement anticipating the New Deal Reforms; then there were the councilar documents of Vatican II; more encyclicals and regional statements of South American Bishops at Medellín and the South African Bishops on apartheid and, in the 1980s, the U.S. Bishops' *Economic Justice for All*. The Catholic Tradition paralleled efforts of other world religions, as demonstrated, for example, by the Protestant Social Gospel movements, by several meetings of the World Council of Churches, and by the Jewish teaching of covenantal justice.

The scholarly presentations examined two major questions: First, what has been the lasting contribution of these writings over the last hundred years? Specifically, how effective have they been in directing economic, political and social thinking by leaders in business, the Church, government and labor, and has there has been any discernible ecumenical impact? And second, today and into the next few decades, what is the unfinished agenda for this tradition of religious writings? A broad selection of representatives were invited from business, labor, government, the Church and the academy to participate in this celebration and to explore the record and future of these writings, namely:

Jean-Yves Calvez, S.J., *Études*, Paris, France; Agostino Cardinal Casaroli, former secretary of state, Vatican; Joan D. Chittister, O.S.B., Benedictine Sisters, Eire, Pennsylvania; M. Shawn Copeland, O.P., Yale Divinity School; Richard T. De George, university distinguished professor of philosophy, University of Kansas; Amitai Etzioni, university professor, George Washington University; J. Bryan Hehir, counselor for social policy, U. S. Catholic Conference, Washington, D.C.; Peter J. Henriot, S.J., former director, Center for Social Concerns, St. Ignatius Church, Lusaka, Zambia; Theodore M. Hesburgh,

C.S.C., president emeritus, University of Notre Dame; Msgr. George G. Higgins, scholar of labor relations, Catholic University of America; Denis E. Hurley, O.M.I., archbishop of Durban, Republic of South Africa; Richard P. McBrien, Crowley-O'Brien-Walter professor of theology, University of Notre Dame; Dennis P. McCann, professor of religious studies, DePaul University; Mark G. McGrath, C.S.C., archbishop of Panama; Michael Novak, senior scholar, American Enterprise Institute, Washington, D.C.; Peter J. Paris, Elmer G. Homrighausen professor of social ethics, Princeton Theological Seminary; William Pfaff, author and political journalist, Paris, France; Paul E. Sigmund, professor of politics, Princeton University.

• • • • •

Publications by the Center include:

Full Value: Cases in Christian Business Ethics
Matter of Dignity: Inquiries into the Humanization of Work
The Judeo-Christian Vision and the Modern Corporation
Co-Creation and Capitalism: John Paul II's "Laborem Exercens"
Catholic Social Teaching and the U.S. Economy
The Common Good and U.S. Capitalism
The Apartheid Crisis
Ethics and the Investment Industry
The Making of an Economic Vision

Articles have appeared in *California Management Review, Business Horizons, Theology Today, Business and Society Review, Horizons, Journal of Business Ethics* and *The Harvard Business Review.*

Part I

Business Stories as Sources of Virtue

"Tell us a story."
"That's only a story."
"Is that story true?"
"Is that the whole story?"

Stories and storytelling have come recently to command a new kind of attention. This interest does not stop with tales but extends to all kinds of narrative and recital, indeed to narrativity itself as distinct from other kinds of discourse. We have long known what a large role fabling, saga, and epic have played in various cultures but we have new reasons for scrutinizing it. On the one hand it begins to dawn on us that a story, a fiction, reveals more than we had thought. One can say that the story tells more than what the storyteller tells. On the other hand we are less assured today as to what we have learned to tell ourselves about life and the world in other kinds of discourse.

Amos N. Wilder

Thus I believe that we have in the vision of Dag Hammarskjöld and that of Martin Luther King a oneness, a wholeness, a holiness not otherwise available to them or to us. Their lives witness to their vision, even as they challenge the depth of our own. So there comes the question, not so much of the suitability of their vision to their own circumstances, but of the justification of our present way of life when held against theirs. Thus theology is drawn by its biographic material to face a challenge not only to its propositions, but also to the selfhood of its practitioners.

James Wm. McClendon, Jr.

1

Narrative is unpretentious in its effect. It does not have, even from God, the dialectical key which will open every door and throw light on the dark passages of history before they have been trodden. It is not, however, without light itself. Pascal drew attention to this light in distinguishing, in his *Memorial*, between the narrated "God of Abraham, Isaac and Jacob" and the God of rational argument, the "God of the philosophers."

Johann Baptist Metz

...the consistency necessary for governing our lives is more a matter of integrity than one of principle. The narratives that provide the pattern of integrity cannot be based on principle, nor are they engaging ways of talking about principles. Rather, such narratives are the ones which allow us to determine how our behavior "fits" within our ongoing pattern.

Stanley Hauerwas and David Burrell

•　•　•　•　•

In 1978 the editors of this volume, Oliver Williams and John Houck, published *Full Value: Cases in Christian Business Ethics*, the inaugural volume of Harper & Row's Experience and Reflection series, which brought narrative theology into dialogue with business practice. We tell this story:

> Once upon a time there once was a father who has two sons. The younger son says , "Father, I want to be my own man. Give me my inheritance early. I'd like to go out and begin my life." So the father gives him the inheritance. The younger son goes out and squanders his money and has a great time. He has all kinds of friends—every-one likes someone with easy money and who has a good time.
>
> Then Jesus goes on to say that, a little time later, the younger son has no money and is literally in the gutter. One day the young son says, "Hey, I don't have to live in the gutter; I can go back and work on my father's farm. The servants there live better than I do now." So he decides to head back home to be a hired hand. "At least I'll have a roof over my head."
>
> Jesus describes this picture of the young son walking down the road. The father, looking out of the farmhouse, spies his son.

The father doesn't know what the son is going to say; he just knows he's coming home. He rejoices and says to the servants, "Kill the fatted calf, prepare for a party. We're going to have a great celebration here."

Now, the elder son comes to the father and says, "Hey, I don't like this. I've been working day in, day out. I am your faithful son, running the operation. You've never killed the fatted calf for me, never had a party like this." The father says, "Your brother has been lost and now has been found."

Our discussion of the meaning is the following:

One important lesson we might learn from the parable is that the Father is merciful, forgiving, and compassionate to a degree beyond our wildest imaginings, and that we ought to try to imitate that sort of love in our lives. Telling this parable, Jesus created the possibility of seeing the world in a whole new way. The very point of the parable was to talk about the familiar secular world in an unfamiliar way, and thus reveal God the Father. Jesus tried to crack the logic of the everyday world and offer a new logic with which to lead one's life. The parable of the prodigal son tells of a rascal who squandered his inheritance and then decided to return home. One would naturally expect the father to be angry and perhaps even insist on some form of retribution. And yet, perhaps to our dismay, the son is the honored guest at a great feast prepared by the father.

Through the story, Jesus suggests to his disciples what his Father is like, and how they might model their lives after God the Father. We might imagine that Jesus asked the disciples after telling the parable: "And what story do you live? Are you like the father who lavished his love on the fallen heir, or are you part of another story with a different logic?" Jesus's use of the image of the Forgiving Father teaches us to allow the Father's love to overflow into our lives, to have a new set of priorities and values. The Scriptures may provide us with a set of images that give us a new vision of our life and circumstances. We "see" with new eyes after being drawn into the parable of the prodigal son.

The Bible may have a decisive influence on a Christian in that it shapes the sort of person he or she is becoming, that is, it has a hand in forming the overall vision of life, the attitudes or dispositions, the convictions, and the intentions of a person. In this light some of the lessons of the parable of the prodigal son might be outlined as follows:

Vision of Life: All humankind is a family and each individual is to be considered as a unique person with his or her distinct contribution. The challenge is to love and care for each other.

Attitudes: The above vision of life disposes us to extend forgiveness to those who have failed. Attitudes of compassion and concern for the downtrodden are engendered.

Convictions: We are confirmed in our fundamental belief that just as our Heavenly Father cares for us, so we must care for each other.

Intentions: We can deliberately choose not to make friends simply for "good contacts," people who will assist in our own personal advancement, but to be present to those who need us and ever alert and ready to extend a hand.

These elements of character formation are not appropriated with one reading of the parable; Christians grow in this way of life by living in the Christian community and being nurtured by the Bible in liturgy, preaching and teaching.

One strength of the parable is that it employs the drama of human conflict to symbolize man's relationship to God. Jesus told the story of a father and his wayward son to dramatize and bring home the way God relates to humankind.

(The above text is from *Full Value: Cases in Christian Business Ethics*, pp. 8-9.)

• • • • •

The business ethicist Oliver Williams and the marketing scholar Patrick Murphy comment on the Johnson & Johnson story:

When an ethics of virtue informs a corporate culture, a shared theory of goods and a common consensus on the hierarchy of goods guides organizational life. The Johnson & Johnson credo expresses this lucidly when it states that the "first responsibility" is to customers and their welfare and the company's last responsibility is to stockholders and their need for profit. The credo offers a vision of how Johnson & Johnson's efforts fit in with the good life that all seek for themselves and their loved ones living in a community. Rules and principles take on meaning, in that they are designed to promote and protect a humane way of life with all its values as they are understood in the community of men and women living and working together. Concern for human welfare, as specified in the hierarchy of values elucidated in the credo, becomes the very glue that holds the firm and its purposes together.

Michael Goldberg, the business consultant-ethicist, tells this story in his essay:

> In the fall of 1982, seven people died when they swallowed Extra Strength Tylenol capsules laced with cyanide. At the time, Tylenol was the top-selling health and beauty aid product in the United States. Its corporate parent, Johnson & Johnson, had built the company reputation on trust and responsibility going back to its founding as an innovator in supplying sterile surgical dressings. Now, J&J was faced with the very real possibility that if it acted in a trustworthy and responsible fashion, it might well lose not only its premier product in the marketplace but a significant slice of its total corporate revenues.

In his essay, Charles McCoy, professor of theological ethics at the Pacific School of Religion and the founding director of both the Center for Ethics and Social Policy, Berkeley, and the Trinity Center for Ethics and Corporate Policy, New York, gives this condensed story:

> Ten senior vice-presidents of a major industrial corporation with over 200 locations scattered over the United States were meeting. The topic for discussion was how to make the corporate code and its ethics more effectively operative throughout the company.

"The real problem, as I see it," Tom was saying, "is whether we do the right thing when issues arise or do what will mean more profit. It's okay to have a code of ethics, but we are first of all in business to make money. If the profit is rolling in, we can afford to put our values into operation."

"I don't think it's that way at all," Bill replied. "We can't make a profit over the long run unless we have a strong culture with value commitments that we are always trying to practice better. One of the main reasons I like working for this company is that I believe we have values and try to build them into what we do."

Chris leaned forward in his seat. "That's what the CEO at Johnson & Johnson was saying in the videotape we saw last week. A corporation has to put the concerns of people first, or society will rebel and pass laws compelling corporations to act in approved ways."

The president of Pittsburgh Theological Seminary, Samuel Calian, a long-time observer of the business scene, suggests "Ten Commandments" for businesspeople:

1. *Treat individuals as sacred;* people are more than means to another's end.

2. *Be generous;* the benefits will exceed the cost in the long term.

3. *Practice moderation;* obsession with winning is dehumanizing and idolatrous.

4. *Disclose mistakes;* confession and restitution are necessary means to restoring ethical character.

5. *Arrange priorities;* have long-range goals and principles in mind.

6. *Keep promises;* trust, confidence, and authenticity are built over a period of time.

7. *Tell the truth;* falsifying information destroys credibility.

8. *Exercise a more inclusive sense of stewardship;* charity does not stop at home but extends throughout our global-oriented society.

9. *Insist on being well informed*; judgment without knowledge is dangerous.

10. *Be profitable without losing your soul in the process*; evaluate your Profit and Loss Statement in light of your trade-offs—a business audit is much more than an accounting of dollars and cents.

Krishna Dhir, professor and director of the School of Business Administration at Pennsylvania State University at Harrisburg, speaking from the Hindu tradition, asks this question:

> If genuine dilemmas are paradoxical and are seldom solved, what is the corporate executive to do? He or she has to be virtuous in decision making. The focus is on the obligations, and on the conflict between individual obligations and social responsibility. The goal has to be not so much to solve moral dilemmas as to *recognize* them.... An example would be helpful. There have been a number of instances where corporations have recalled products from the marketplace in the interests of the consumer and society. The recalls of Tylenol by Johnson & Johnson and the Rely product by Procter and Gamble are examples of corporate decisions exhibiting uncommon virtue. In these instances, the executives decided on actions which did not necessarily fulfill their obligations to the stockholders, employees, and other parties. However, they acted to protect human welfare and save lives. They knew they faced a genuine moral dilemma. They did not solve the dilemma. They did not fulfill all their obligations. They opted to fulfill the obligation of social responsibility. They made this choice through enlightened wisdom, and they resolved the moral dilemma effectively.

One

The Ethics of Virtue: A Moral Theory for Business*

Oliver F. Williams and Patrick E. Murphy

The field of marketing ethics is a burgeoning one. Although the systematic study of it is only just over twenty years old, recent emphasis on the subject has grown dramatically. Fueled by ethical transgressions by marketing managers such as the widely reported events surrounding the defense contractors and the infant formula industry in developing countries, the examination of ethical behavior by marketers has received increasing attention by scholars. (For reviews of this work, see Murphy and Laczniak 1981; Murphy and Pridgen 1991.)

This article proposes that the ethics of virtue is a very relevant theory for improving the ethical conduct of marketers. Although this ethical theory has received only modest attention by marketing writers to date, it holds much promise for effectively examining and promoting ethical behavior. The point here is that much of the behavior cited as exemplary in the corporate world, for example the Tylenol decision by Johnson & Johnson or the Rely decision by Procter and Gamble,[1] is not sufficiently explained as just principled action. Rather, what made the top management of these firms corporate heroes in the eyes of many is that they exhibited uncommon virtue in maintaining allegiance to their principles. This was demonstrated, for example, in the *courage* to act to protect human welfare even in the midst of incomplete information and in the *integrity* and *humility* displayed in communicating with consumers about possible difficulties with a product. Before we discuss the theory of virtue in depth, we examine the ethical theories developed in moral philosophy that have been applied to marketing issues.

*A slightly different version of this paper was printed in the *Journal of Macromarketing*, Spring 1990.

Ethical Theory Applied to Marketing

It is generally accepted that there are two classes of ethical theory, both of which yield principles for action: teleology and deontology. Useful definitions of each are proposed by Kimmel (1988):

> A teleological theory of ethics holds an action as morally right or obligatory if it or the rule under which it falls will produce the greatest possible balance of good over evil.

> The term deontology has evolved from the Greek *deon* (duty) and *logos* (science and reason), suggesting that certain acts are to be viewed as morally right or obligatory not because of their effects on human welfare, but rather because they keep a promise, show gratitude, demonstrate loyalty to an unconditional command, and the like.

The most widely known teleological theory is utilitarianism, espoused by John Stuart Mill (Piest 1957). Two subcategories of utilitarianism—rule and act—are recognized. Ethical egoism falls within this theory. There are also two general approaches to deontology: duty-based theories, such as Kant's "categorical imperative" (Wolff 1985) and Ross's (1930) *prima facie* duties, and rights-based approach, whose best known proponent is John Rawls (1971).

Recognizing the crucial need to formulate principles that will guide the decision maker in establishing priorities among the various "goods" to be sought and "evils" to be avoided, marketing scholars have drawn on the deontological and utilitarian theories. Murphy and Laczniak (1981) summarize these theories and state that "ethics is fundamentally a matter of moral philosophy" (p. 252). Laczniak (1983) reviews three significant deontological frameworks proposed by Ross (1930), Garrett (1966) and Rawls (1971). He then applies their major principles to problems in marketing ethics. In their empirical examination of management behavior, Fritzsche and Becker (1984), drawing on the work of Cavanagh, Moberg and Velasquez (1981), suggest that there are three prominent ethical theories—utilitarianism, rights, and justice (the latter two fall within the deontological theories).

Three major attempts to develop a theory of marketing ethics also use the teleology-deontology dichotomy as background for their work. Ferrell and Gresham (1985) discuss utilitarianism, the rights principle, and the justice principle as the components of the individual factors construct in their contingency framework for examining marketing ethics. Hunt and Vitell's (1986) article on the theory of marketing ethics contained an extensive discussion of moral philosophy, and they also employ these two ethical theories. They conclude, however, that: "any positive theory of ethics must account for both the deontological and teleological aspects of the evaluation process" (p. 7). Most recently, Ferrell, Gresham and Fraedrich (1989) reviewed these moral philosophies before proposing their "synthesis model" of ethical decision making.

The writings of Robin and his colleagues have built primarily on these two theories. Robin and Reidenbach (1988) develop their use of deontological and utilitarian theories onto the matrix of Miller's living system hierarchy. Robin and others (1989) evaluate corporate codes of conduct using deontological and utilitarian standards.

In a 1987 article in the *Journal of Marketing*, Robin and Reidenbach offer an insightful proposal for developing an ethical corporate culture in a business organization. Relying primarily on the widely used ethical theories of deontology and utilitarianism, this article presents a good example of the prevailing thinking in the field; therefore, their work, which highlights a theory of virtue rather than one of the principles-based theories, will be cited in arguing the case for a new approach to structuring an ethical corporate culture.

The Meaning of Social Responsibility and Ethics

Exactly what role do ethics play in determining a corporate culture?[2] Robin and Reidenbach (1987) are aware that the philosophers are not in complete agreement on this point. Consequently, they chart out their understanding of ethics and social responsibility and demonstrate how these might be incorporated into a business culture. Following much of the "business and society" literature, they make a distinction between social responsibility and business ethics:

> Corporate social responsibility is related to the social contract between business and the society in which it operates....Business ethics, in contrast, requires that the organization or individual behave in accordance with the carefully thought-out rules of moral philosophy (p. 45).

The assumption is made that a business culture ought to reflect the dominant ethical values present in our capitalistic democracy. Further, it is assumed that "two of the most popular ethical traditions," deontology and utilitarianism, are the best means of reflecting the ethics of democratic capitalism. Two principles are enunciated to guide corporate culture. First, marketing activities that have a foreseeable and potentially serious impact on individuals ought to be regulated by the values of deontological reasoning. Second, for all marketing exchanges that do not have foreseeable serious consequences for individuals, the arguments of utilitarianism seem appropriate.

Both deontology, with its concern for individual "rights," and utilitarianism, with its social focus on "the greatest good for the greatest number," have a role to play in adjudicating ethical quandaries. In addition, the authors offer a third ethical theory, "virtue ethics," which, according to them, counsels that "neither excessiveness nor deficiency in performance would be acceptable. Rather, "a 'golden mean' of performance" should be sought (p. 51). Moderation or "prudence" is highlighted.

Once an organization has a mission statement, an appreciation for the rules of deontology and utilitarianism, and a cognizance of the import of family values (which Robin and Reidenbach propose are similar to those held by organizations—Table 1 in their article), the firm's managers then formulate core ethical values that will become the organization's hallmark. For example, if the mission statement highlights a strong customer orientation, the authors articulate the core value as follows: "Treat customers with respect, concern, and honesty, the way you yourself would want to be treated or the way you would want your family treated" (p. 55). Core values guide marketing plans and inform day-to-day practice.

What a Theory of Virtue Might Provide

When analyzing some of the difficult cases that have captured the widespread attention of the American public, such as the Tylenol or Rely product recall decisions, what becomes clear is that business experts, using one or the other theories of principles, were quite divided on the "right" response to the crisis. Even at its best, moral reasoning does not yield unambiguous results. A case could have been, and was made, for *not* withdrawing the Tylenol and Rely products. To be sure, the principles provided by the ethical theories offer some guidance to the decision makers as they seek the right choices between the conflicting goods (goods here refer not to products but alternative choices). But in the face of divided opinion and the fear of making a mistake, some individuals have the ability to see what to do, rise to the occasion and muster the courage to act; these people often become our heroes. It may be that a theory of virtue best explains these human strengths and can assist in cultivating organizations that foster their development.

Most often today, discussions of virtue ethics in the literature are inadequate. The Aristotelian ethics of virtue, as retrieved in the work of the contemporary philosopher Alasdair MacIntyre, offers much promise. MacIntyre defines *virtue* as "an acquired human quality the possession and exercise of which tends to enable us to achieve those goods which are internal to practices and the lack of which effectively prevents us from achieving any such good" (MacIntyre 1981, p. 178). The point here is that character or virtue is *acquired*; these human capacities or qualities are cultivated by choices and by the environments within which we live and work. An equally important point in the definition is that acting virtuously truly is its own reward, that is, while acting virtuously may indeed yield good results (such as increased market share for Tylenol), virtuous decision makers act primarily to be true to themselves. What MacIntyre is getting at here is that there are a range of goods (goods *internal* to practices) which are valued not because of their utilitarian significance in that they yield desired outcomes, but because they are a part of what it means to be a person. The young student who exercises great discipline and masters a musical instrument may indeed get an "A" in the course (a good external and secondary to the practice), but the significant reward is the ability to enjoy good music at a new and higher level (a good internal to the practice). The claim is that virtues are what makes life interesting and worth living. Some of the virtues highlighted for the professions by one ethicist advocating a theory of virtue include perseverance, courage, integrity, compassion, candor, fidelity, prudence, public-spiritedness, justice and humility (May 1984).

When an ethics of virtue informs a corporate culture, a shared theory of goods and a common consensus on the hierarchy of goods guides organizational life. The Johnson & Johnson credo expresses this lucidly when it states that the "first responsibility" is to customers and their welfare and the company's last responsibility is to stockholders and their

Our Credo

We believe our first responsiblity is to the doctors, nurses and patients,
to mothers and fathers and all others who use our products and services.
In meeting their needs everything we do must be of high quality.
We must constantly strive to reduce our costs
in order to maintain reasonable prices.
Customers' orders must be serviced promptly and accurately.
Our suppliers and distributors must have an opportunity
to make a fair profit.

We are responsible to our employees,
the men and women who work with us throughout the world.
Everyone must be considered as an individual.
We must respect their dignity and recognize their merit.
They must have a sense of security in their jobs.
Compensation must be fair and adequate,
and working conditions clean, orderly and safe.
We must be mindful of ways to help our employees fulfill
their family responsibilities.
Employees must feel free to make suggestions and complaints.
There must be equal opportunity for employment, development
and advancement for those qualified.
We must provide competent management,
and their actions must be just and ethical.

We are responsible to the communities in which we live and work
and to the world community as well.
We must be good citizens — support good works and charities
and bear our fair share of taxes.
We must encourage civic improvements and better health and education.
We must maintain in good order
the property we are privileged to use
protecting the environment and natural resources.

Our final responsibility is to our stockholders.
Business must make a sound profit.
We must experiment with new ideas.
Research must be carried on, innovative programs developed
and mistakes paid for.
New equipment must be purchased, new facilities provided
and new products launched.
Reserves must be created to provide for adverse times.
When we operate according to these principles,
the stockholders should realize a fair return.

Johnson & Johnson

need for profit. The credo offers a vision of how Johnson & Johnson's efforts fit in with the good life that all seek for themselves and their loved ones living in a community. Rules and principles take on meaning, in that they are designed to promote and protect a humane way of life with all its values as they are understood in the community of men and women living and working together. Concern for human welfare, as specified in the hierarchy of values elucidated in the credo, becomes the very glue that holds the firm and its purposes together.

The importance of this discussion of virtue ethics may be informed further by returning to the Robin and Reidenbach article. Following a familiar pattern, the rationale offered as to why marketers ought to respond to society's demands is that, if they do not, further regulations likely will be enacted. Why, then, use the values of the family as a yardstick for business organizations? Is the only reason political (that is, to forestall the restrictive regulation that angry consumers might demand) or are there moral reasons (Frederick 1986; Epstein 1987)? Clearly there are, says the theory of virtue, because, on some level, the values or virtues that prevail in family life must permeate all of society if we are to avoid being overcome by greed and corruption.

The case of Nestlé's sale of infant formula in developing countries is cited by Robin and Reidenbach (1987) as an illustration of how deontological arguments prevailed over utilitarian arguments; in the face of consumer pressure, the company finally "agreed to follow the dictates of the World Health Organization (WHO) Code" (p. 50). It is true that the final resolution was company adherence to the WHO Code, and it is probable that the force of moral arguments aroused the citizenry to consumer boycotts and other pressures which finally forced the company to comply. Although compelling moral reasons may have marshalled the opposition to Nestlé, these reasons are not captured clearly in the trade-off model of the two theories of principles (deontological and utilitarian) presented. A theory of virtue may provide deeper insight into the problem at Nestlé and some direction for the future.

Nestlé's failure was not that they did not *know* deontological reasoning and ethical core values; probably it can be safely assumed that management in the Swiss-based company was quite familiar with this scenario, if only because they had been hearing it from their activist opponents for almost six years before agreeing to conform to the WHO Code. Stressing the freedom of choice of consumers, Nestlé management never seemed to give much weight to the fact that most Third

World mothers did not have the capacity to make an informed choice about infant formula or to use the product safely. Even after it became clear that consumers were using the product incorrectly, Nestlé still did not see the issue as its problem.

Unlike the credo-inspired corporate culture of fidelity of Johnson & Johnson, Nestlé seemed to be operating with the outdated notion of *caveat emptor* (let the buyer beware). When the virtue of fidelity serves as the glue of a business organization, there is a promise by the business to its public that every effort will be made to look out for human welfare within the limits of its operation. The Johnson & Johnson Tylenol withdrawal was not so much a matter of telling the truth (principled action) as it was of being true to its promise (virtuous action). Nestlé management took its stand on freedom (principled action) but seemed to lack those qualities of character (such as prudence) which help orient one to the appropriate principle for the reality in question. The use of deontological reasoning makes it clear that Nestlé had a blind spot, but this approach itself is not the remedy for the malady. The ethics of virtue help make this apparent blindness understandable and point toward its cure.

The Ethics of Virtue

The ethics of virtue assume that being human entails living in community and developing certain virtues or skills required for a humane life with others. By trial and error, human reason arrives at certain core virtues for community living—such character traits as honesty, truthfulness, compassion, loyalty and justice. Various capacities have highlighted different eras; for example, the classical virtues discussed by Plato, Aristotle and Cicero were discussed as prudence, justice, courage and temperance. To be sure, the world view of Aristotle and his time is far from our own, but the theory of virtue still has much relevance.

In the ethics of virtue, or character, such traits or moral virtues as compassion, loyalty and justice shape a person's vision. There is some truth to the saying that "only the good person knows the good"; only a person who has developed the moral virtues, who is compassionate, just, and so on, will perceive the tough moral dilemmas and make correct judgments. Of course, these are not new ideas. Aristotle, particularly in the *Nicomachaen Ethics* (Irwin 1985) and the *Politics*, has much to say to our times:

...the same things do not seem sweet to a man in a fever and a healthy man—nor hot to a weak man and one in good condition. The same happens in other cases. But in all such matters that which appears to the good man is thought to be really so (Bk.X, ch. 5, 1176a).

For Aristotle, virtues make a person good, and virtue entails affectivity; affectivity influences one's ability to "see" the moral dimensions of a situation:

...for to feel delight and pain rightly or wrongly has no small effect on our actions (Bk. II, ch. 2, 1105a).

Affectivity, however, is learned behavior:

Hence we ought to have been brought up in a particular way from our youth, as Plato says, so as both to delight in and to be pained by the things that we ought; for this is right education (Bk. II, ch. 2, 1104b).

In a theory of virtue, the rightness or wrongness of an action, such as a TV advertisement, would be tied to how that ad would be likely to shape the viewers. Moral virtue is understood to be essential to making good assessments and judgments, that is, without having cultivated generosity, compassion, forgiveness, and so on, one will not "see" all that is there. With moral virtue, the intellect is affectively qualified in that it is attentive to certain features of experience that it might otherwise miss or undervalue.

A theory of virtue enables business organizations to develop consciously their own ethical corporate culture (see Williams and Houck 1978; Williams 1984). A business organization can so shape people that they do not "see" the ethical dimensions of the professional world. When efficiency and productivity are the only values reinforced in the organization, people slowly are molded to do whatever will "get the job done" without adverting to broader considerations. Treating people functionally may gradually constrict their perspective so that their "world" is essentially functional. This can affect the features of their experience to which they attend and, consequently, how they describe situations. For example, a long-time employee who is not performing adequately in his or her present position may be seen as "an incompetent who must be fired" or as "a person in the wrong position who must be reassigned." To a large extent, it depends upon whether the cultural distortions of functionality and rationality dominate, or whether sensitivity to human dignity is shaping one's vision.

Most attempts to integrate the ethical dimension into the corporate culture concentrate on the two major theories of obligation without adverting to the integrative possibilities of the more comprehensive theory of virtue. What constitutes "good" and "ethical" marketing? In the commonly employed theories of obligation, the deontological and the utilitarian, this question is answered by referring to the standards of right and wrong, where rightness or wrongness are determined by rules and principles or by some assessment of the consequences of a practice. In the theory of virtue, however, the central questions are, What sort of person am I shaping? and What sort of organization am I shaping? by this proposed decision or policy. Thus, the perspective of this ethical system is that all rules and principles are, at root, an attempt to preserve a humane way of life; our most fundamental task in ethics today, therefore, is not concerned primarily with analyzing situations so that one can make the right decisions, but rather with reflecting on what constitutes the good life. The moral life is not so much a matter of thinking clearly as it is a way of "seeing" the world. The Johnson & Johnson credo is a good example of an attempt to provide a humane world view for all constituencies.

The problem at Nestlé was not that decision makers were not thinking clearly but rather that managers were adverting to the wrong features of their experience. This is a problem explicitly addressed by the formation of an ethical corporate culture, for the culture does indeed shape one's vision. Underpinned by a theory of virtue, an ethical corporate culture, through an ingrained set of habits and perspectives, trains all those in its purview to see things in a certain way and hence is likely to predispose them toward ethical behavior.

In a theory of virtue, there is much attention to role models. The insight here is that being an ethical person is not simply an analytical and rational matter. It takes virtuous people to make right decisions, and virtue is learned by doing. To teach ethics, Aristotle discussed the lives of obviously good Athenians. One learned the right thing to do by observing good people and by doing what they do:

> ...but the virtues we get by first exercising them, as also happens in the case of the arts as well. For the things we have to learn before we can do them, we learn by doing them, e.g. men become builders by

building and lyre-players by playing the lyre; so too we become just by doing just acts, temperate by doing temperate acts, brave by doing brave acts (Bk. II, ch. 1, 1103a).

The companies acclaimed for their ethical corporate culture usually can trace their heritage to one or several founders who were intent on managing an organization that respected human dignity and insisted on a humane way of life. Founders of such companies as Johnson & Johnson and Hewlett-Packard shaped their organizations so that they embodied the values and virtues that proved personally rewarding. The way of life in the company was not a result of a core values analysis or a code of conduct; rather, these vehicles were a later attempt to spell out exactly what was at the heart of this corporate culture already under way. For example, Bill Hewlett and Dave Packard did not formulate their company values in writing until after twenty years of operation. Only then, to ensure that the culture would not be lost as the founders became more removed from the expanding workforce, did top management draw up a statement of corporate values, initiate training seminars in the "HP Way," and install accountability procedures (Williams 1986).

For companies without a heritage of the Hewlett-Packard or Johnson & Johnson type, Robin and Reidenbach (1987) have provided some helpful practical steps to begin to develop an ethical corporate culture. They have not, however, delineated an ethical theory which can offer an account of what is happening in such a culture; the contention here is that the ethics of virtue is such a theory.

Although principles clearly are essential to help guide the ethical choices of the decision maker, "principles without traits are impotent" in the words of a renowned philosopher (Frankena 1974, p. 65). Principles, whether they be of a deontological or utilitarian variety, need a context, a vision of what constitutes the good life. For example, the principle "be caring" would be understood one way by Ivan Boesky and quite another way by John Phelan, Jr., chairman of the board of the New York Stock Exchange and a leading exponent of ethical conduct on the "Street." The same principle would have different meanings for persons with divergent horizons of interpretation. The principle was designed to preserve a humane way of life in community, but it will function only in that fashion if its user has a vision of such a community in mind.

Actually, it is ingenuous to suggest the family as the horizon for interpreting moral principles for a business organization (Robin & Reidenbach 1987). The family unit is the one place where our humanity is evoked and virtuous relationships are almost always in place, at least as an ideal. The sense of what constitutes caring or honesty or most other virtues is easily grasped by looking to the family. A theory of virtue highlights the moral obligation to bring some of the virtues we all experience in the family into the workplace, as Hewlett-Packard has done. This is just another way of saying that a business organization ought to be a humane community. To be sure, one must be reasonable and there is no iron-clad method of determining how much caring is required, but virtuous people can make prudent decisions.

Johnson & Johnson: Some Further Reflections

As noted above, one company often singled out for its "well developed system of core values" is Johnson & Johnson. Although this assessment is accurate, it is more important to ask: From where do these values emanate, and how are they supported and sustained? The theory of virtue sheds light and offers an understanding of exemplary corporate cultures.

From its founding a century ago by three brothers, Johnson & Johnson has grown to a multinational firm with sales of over $7 billion. The company operates 160 businesses in more than 50 countries. The hallmarks of the organization are that it is managed with a long-run view, decentralization is a key management philosophy, and the Johnson & Johnson credo guides its business activities. Many of the phrases in the credo delineate what this company interprets as its hierarchy of "goods" and how the organization shapes the values of its stakeholders. The credo was instituted first in 1945 and has been revised twice since then. At the request of the then chairman, James Burke, the credo was "challenged" in the 1970s by Johnson & Johnson managers and the consequence was basically an affirmation of it. This exercise did result in a new 1979 credo with slight rewording of the previous one.

The company's reaction to the Tylenol poisonings of 1982 are viewed by many observers as representing the type of responsible behavior that all companies should exemplify. The firms's recall of the Tylenol capsules was a result of the culture in place at Johnson & Johnson for a long time and was more than just clear reasoning about the company values. One senior Johnson & Johnson executive expressed the firm's perspective well when he said, "We never really thought we had much of a choice in the matter of the recall. Our code of conduct (credo) was such a way of life in the firm that our employees, including me, would have been scandalized had we taken another course. We never seriously considered avoiding the costly recall" (Nash 1988). The Johnson & Johnson decision was determined largely, then, by its way of seeing the problem, and its ingrained habits (not by reasoning about core ethical values). Virtues such as courage, compassion and lucidity, long operative in the organization, came to the foreground in the quandary over the Tylenol crisis.[3]

A second illustration of Johnson & Johnson's virtuous corporate culture is in the decision concerning operations in South Africa. After a careful moral analysis, the company decided to maintain its plants and investment there. Several constituencies in the United States have pressed strongly for disinvestment, but the firm disagrees on moral grounds and has not yielded to the pressure. Because of Johnson & Johnson's ethical corporate culture and long-standing commitment to humane values, their response has not been criticized, for the most part, even by those who justifiably hold a contrary position. Often it is in those cases where a theory of principle does not yield an answer compelling to all that a virtuous organization is readily apparent. Human strengths keep the argument over principles from taking a destructive tack; humility, intellectual caution and good faith are virtues that preserve a humane community even while the dispute continues.

A third example pertains to a successful advertising campaign that ran a decade ago for Johnson & Johnson Baby Oil (Baby, Baby! Turn on the Tan with Johnson's). At that time there was little concern about the sun's harmful effects on the skin. A medical acquaintance of a Johnson & Johnson executive pointed out initial evidence that tanning might be harmful and that, since baby oil increases the rate of the burning and tanning process, the product indirectly could be harmful. After further investigation, Johnson & Johnson executives found this was the case and dropped the campaign. As the executive who made the decision stated, "It simply would be wrong to entice people to harm themselves" (Nash 1988, p. 98). To be sure, this was principled action, but action brought to the fore by the virtues of courage and integrity.

These examples convey how one company's behavior can be understood in the light of a theory of virtue. The pervasiveness of the Johnson & Johnson credo throughout the organization and the consistent ethical focus by managers show how moral reasoning is shaped by a virtuous environment and how that, in turn, influences managerial decision making.

Marketing and the Theory of Virtue

The theory of virtue has a bearing on the type of marketing mix decisions a company and manager makes. Implications for product, pricing, channel and promotional decisions emanate from this theory. For product decisions, the theory of virtue would emphasize the product's impact upon consumers' lives. Does the product pose potential harm to the consumer? For certain products, an especially vulnerable segment may be harmed. What about targeting cigarettes to young women or blacks, alcohol to young men, pornography to juveniles? In these cases is there not a strong possibility of eroding the formation of virtue in a young life and of stunting public spiritedness and citizenship in the future? The theory of virtue thus highlights the need for marketers to consider questions of how consumers are being affected by each product. We suggest that marketers should not sell products that retard character or virtue development.

The pricing area is one that has received little attention from ethics scholars (Kehoe 1985). The theories of obligation as well as the theory of virtue would require marketers to place price in a perspective understandable to the potential market. For example, confusing airline fares and auto company financing plans may not meet the moral requirements of pricing products. Yet, complex fares may be viewed as more ethical (that is, virtuous) than a single monopoly price charged to consumers (as happened prior to deregulation), and multiple financing plans could be more ethical than a simple but very expensive, one. Furthermore, the theory of virtue would emphasize the price-value trade-off about which consumers are concerned when entering into the exchange process for products. For example, clear delineation of list price, discounted price and exceptions by retailers would embrace the spirit of the theory of virtue. It is interesting to note that these areas are being studied by the Better Business Bureau and a group of influential retailers (*Avertising Age* 1989).

The channel of distribution can present many ethical dilemmas for marketers because of the multiple intermediaries and the complex relationships among channel members that often exist. The theory of virtue would place priority on honesty and cooperation in dealings between channel members rather than on the coercion and conflict often cited. Furthermore, the move toward relational (that is, relationship-based) exchanges in the channel should be more conducive to virtuous behavior (Gundlach and Murphy 1990). Larger organizations in the channel, which are growing in number, would not attempt to coerce smaller ones unduly if they were to follow this theory.

The theory of virtue also can be applied to the promotional element of the marketing mix. For personal selling, the emphasis would be on positive character traits such as honesty, integrity, justice and prudence. These are undervalued by companies that want aggressive, high pressure, short-term, results-oriented salespeople. Managers wishing to employ the theory of virtue might investigate how sales training and positive customer experiences can enhance sales results. The relationship that salespersons have with consumers would be shaped also by the theory of virtue. Consumers would be viewed as partners in the exchange process and not as potential adversaries or pawns in the sales game. It appears that industrial salespeople often take a more "virtuous" stance because their relationship with customers is ongoing.

Advertising ethics also would take a different approach with an application of the theory of virtue. For example, a recent article on ethics in advertising examined how one should make a moral appraisal of advertising (Lee 1987). The literature is divided among those who believe that persuasive advertising is (a) moral so long as it promotes a useful or essential product; (b) never good; and (c) good so long as it does not affect individual autonomy. However, none of these positions adequately reflects the theory of virtue which is concerned with how the person is being shaped or how the consumer's character may be formed by the advertisement.

The theory of virtue would demand that managers think about how advertising influences its recipients. There is growing concern by some professionals that through marketing, and especially advertising, people are being shaped and formed in inappropriate and perhaps harmful ways. For example, consider the views of psychiatrist Thomas Radecki, research director for the National Coalition on Television Violence, who argues that restrictions must be placed on the marketing of war toys on television. He cites substantial studies indicating that the massive promotion of war toys "encourages violent ways of interacting with the world." More hitting, selfishness and cruelty to animals are evidenced in children exposed to such television, according to Radecki. Although this is still a controversial finding, it highlights an increasing focus on the influences that shape character or virtues in the young.

Today, a whole new set of demands flow from a broader understanding of ethics, and these demands will pose a continuing quandary for marketers unless there is a genuine comprehension of the critics' positions. For example, advocates of less aggression, violence and sex in advertising have an understanding of what constitutes "good" and "ethical" advertising that is well grounded in the ethics of virtue. It is in the marketer's interest to be familiar with this approach to ethics.

International marketing ethics are compounded by cultural, religious, social and language differences, but the theory of virtue offers universal traits that can be applied across cultures. Exceptions obviously exist, but treating consumers with compassion, respect and integrity would seem to transcend international boundaries. For example, Dow Corning conducts "ethical audits" at its plants and sales offices worldwide to make sure that the company's values statement is interpreted consistently everywhere. Likewise, many of the suspect practices of international marketers, such as product dumping and inadequate product usage information for infant formula, clearly violate the precepts of the theory of virtue.

Conclusion

This chapter has summarized how ethical theory has influenced the marketing ethics literature. The major premise is that ethical analysis could be improved with a focus on the theory of virtue. Further, the chapter has spelled out in detail what the theory of virtue is and how it can provide a central position in the ethical development of marketers. It shows also how certain companies known for ethical behavior, in particular Johnson & Johnson, are much better understood in the light of a theory of virtue than from the perspectives of other philosophical theories. The chapter also includes a discussion of how the theory of virtue could influence the marketing strategies used by companies.

Future research could build on the foundation developed here. An in-depth comparison of this theory with deontological and teleological theories could be used to evaluate specific marketing actions. Further study is needed to determine how best the theory of virtue might complement other ethical theories (Beauchamp 1982, p. 163). Finally, this traditional ethical theory needs to be evaluated relative to other ethical approaches (Kohlberg 1969; Rest 1986) to see if they add specificity to this broad notion. The theory of virtue has much applicability to marketing ethics. Even though more work needs to be done, the theory provides needed answers to the debate concerning a more ethical marketing system.

Notes

1. "The possible connection between tampons and toxic shock became known in 1980, when several deaths led to the withdrawal of the high-absorbency Rely brand tampons made by Procter & Gamble. In 1982, a panel of scientists reported that women 15 to 24 years old were at greatest risk of contracting the disease," *New York Times*, June 29, 1984, p. 13.

2. A common definition of corporate culture, and one to which we subscribe, is offered by Uttal (1983): the system of shared values (what is important) and beliefs (how things work) that interact with a company's people, organizational structures, and control systems to produce behavioral norms (how we do things around here).

3. The most recent information indicates that the Tylenol brand was ranked the highest in terms of quality by a consumer study (Lipman 1989), and held the largest market share (27% versus 12% for second place) in the pain-remedy category (Deveny 1990).

Bibliography

Advertising Age, "Retail Code Worth the Price," September 25, 1989.

Beauchamp, Tom L., *Philosophical Ethics: An Introduction to Moral Philosophy* (New York: McGraw-Hill, 1982).

Cavanagh, G.F., Moberg, D.J., and Velasquez, M., "The Ethics of Organizational Politics," *Academy of Management Review*, 6 (July 1981), 363-374.

Deveny, Kathleen, "Painkiller Ads Strive to Give Foes Headaches," *Wall Street Journal*, January 23, 1990, B1.

Epstein, Edwin, "The Corporate Social Policy Process: Beyond Business Ethics, Corporate Social Responsibility, and Corporate Social Responsiveness," *California Management Review*, 29 (Spring 1987), 99-114.

Ferrell, O.C., and Gresham, L., "A Contingency Framework for Understanding Ethical Decision Making in Marketing," *Journal of Marketing*, 49 (Summer 1985), 87-96.

Ferrell, O. C., Gresham, L. G., and Fraedrich, J., "A Synthesis of Ethical Decision Models for Marketing," *Journal of Macromarketing*, 9 (Fall 1989), 55-64.

Frankena, William K., *Ethics*, 2nd ed. (Englewood Cliffs, NJ: Prentice-Hall, 1974).

Frederick, William, "Toward CSR2: Why Ethical Analysis Is Indispensable and Unavoidable in Corporate Affairs," *California Management Review*, 28 (Winter 1986), 126-41, 152-53.

Fritzsche, D., and Becker, H., "Linking Management Behavior to Ethical Philosophy—An Empirical Investigation," *Academy of Management Journal*, 27, 1 (1984), 166-75.

Garrett, Thomas, *Business Ethics* (Englewood Cliffs, NJ: Prentice-Hall, 1966).

Gundlach, Gregory T., and Murphy, Patrick E., "Ethical and Legal Foundations of Exchange," paper presented to Winter American Marketing Association Educators' Conference, 1990.

Hunt, S.D., and Vitell, S., "A General Theory of Marketing Ethics," *Journal of Macromarketing*, 6 (Spring 1986), 5-16.

Irwin, Terence, trans. *Nicomachean Ethics*, by Aristotle (Indianapolis, IN: Hackett, 1985).

Kehoe, William J., "Ethics, Price Fixing, and the Management of Price Strategy," *Marketing Ethics: Guidelines for Managers*, G.R. Laczniak and P.E. Murphy, eds. (Lexington, MA: Lexington Books, 1985), 71-83.

Kimmel, Allan J., *Ethics and Values in Applied Social Research* (Beverly Hills, CA: Sage, 1988).

Kohlberg, L., "State and Sequence: The Cognitive Developmental Approach to Socialization," *Handbook of Socialization Theory and Research*, D.A. Goslin, ed. (Chicago: Rand McNally, 1969), 347-480.

Laczniak, G.R., "Frameworks for Analyzing Marketing Ethics," *Journal of Macromarketing*, 5 (Spring 1983), 7-17.

Lee, Kam Hon, "The Informative and Persuasive Functions of Advertising: A Moral Appraisal—A Further Comment," *Journal of Business Ethics*, 6 (January 1987), 55-57.

Lipman, Joanne, "Top Brands Rank Low in Study of Quality," *Wall Street Journal*, (June 6, 1989), B5.

MacIntyre, Alasdair, *After Virtue*, (Notre Dame, IN: University of Notre Dame Press, 1981).

Murphy, Patrick E., and Pridgen, M. Dee, "Ethical and Legal Issues in Marketing," *Advances in Marketing and Public Policy*, 2 (1991), 185-244.

Nash, Laura L., "Johnson & Johnson's Credo," in *Corporate Ethics: A Prime Business Asset*, The Business Roundtable, ed. (February 1988), 77-104.

Piest, Oskar, ed., *John Stewart Mill, Utilitarianism* (New York: Macmillan, 1957).

Rawls, John, *A Theory of Justice* (Cambridge, MA: Harvard University Press, 1971).

Rest, James R., *Moral Development: Advances in Research and Theory* (New York: Praeger, 1986).

Robin, Donald, Giallourakis, Michael, David, Fred R., and Moritz, Thomas E., *Business Horizons*, 32 (January-February 1989), 66-73.

Robin, Donald P., and Reidenbach, R. Eric, "Social Responsibility, Ethics, and Marketing Strategy: Closing the Gap between Concept and Application," *Journal of Marketing*, 51 (January 1987), 44-58.

"A Framework For Analyzing Ethical Issues in Marketing," *Business and Professional Ethics Journal*, 5, 2 (1988), 3-22.

Ross, William David, *The Right and the Good* (Oxford: Clarendon Press, 1930).

Uttal, B., "The Corporate Culture Vultures," *Fortune*, (October 1983), 66-72.

Williams, Oliver F., "Who Cast the First Stone?" *Harvard Business Review*, 62, 5 (1984), 151-60.

"Can Business Ethics Be Theological? What Athens Can Learn from Jerusalem," *Journal of Business Ethics*, 5 (December 1986), 473-484.

Williams, Oliver F., and Houck, John W., *Full Value: Cases in Christian Business Ethics* (San Francisco: Harper and Row, 1978).

Wolff, Robert Paul, ed., *Foundations of the Metaphysics of Morals* by Immanuel Kant (New York: Macmillan, 1985).

Two

Corporate Culture and the Corporate Cult

Michael Goldberg

The Era of Human Capital

As U.S. business enters the last decade of the century, its corporate watchword might well be "*The era of 'human capital' is upon us.*"[1] The structural barriers of the past that protected companies—geography, regulation, technology and scale—are all breaking down. Where the strategic question of the '80s was, Where best to compete? the question for the '90s is, Who can compete best?[2] Thus, whereas in the decade just past, the agenda was dominated by financial matters such as economic forecasts and stock values, business strategies in the coming decade will be governed more and more by such matters of corporate culture as corporate vision and corporate values.

That '90s phenomenon may well imply another: At the end of the twentieth century, some U.S. corporations may constitute the closest thing our society has to community. Such companies form communities of their members by providing them with common goals, common procedures for attaining those goals, and common standards for marking success and failure. Unlike most other associations in contemporary American life, ranging from mens' clubs to marriages, the corporate community's existence depends on neither "mutual admiration" nor a "spirit of volunteerism"; businesspeople who find themselves in a corporate setting are not necessarily nor even primarily together because they like each other. Instead, what bonds such people to one another is "a sense of reliance on one another toward a common cause."[3]

Such talk of joint reliance in pursuit of a common cause may call to mind medieval sagas of sacred quests for holy grails. No wonder. For some corporations hold out to their members a community of a particular kind: in fundamental ways, the community they present is a *religious* one.

Although speaking of a corporation as a religious community may at first sound shocking, we find among the earliest manifestations of corporations just that—namely, such corporate bodies as monasteries and bishoprics. Thus, St. Benedict, for instance, wished to form a religious institution that was virtually self-contained, a kind of miniature society. Indeed, the very word "corporation" springs from the root *corpus*, signifying a *"body sharing a common purpose in a common name."*[4]

Closer to our own time, several observers have noted the key role that corporate cultures play in shaping the attitudes and actions of those who inhabit them. But few, if any, commentators have noticed a kindred concept closely related to culture: *cult.* For both cult and culture trace their roots back to a common etymological ancestor, *colere*, meaning "to cultivate" or "cherish." Indeed, for many late twentieth century Americans, the corporate *cultus* is more cherished, more venerated, than any other modern institution—including their churches and synagogues. The corporation and its cult not only help construct the basic reality of their lives *à la* Geertz but *à la* Tillich; they help furnish those lives with such "ultimate concerns" as meaning, vision and values. Consequently, for Americans such as these, i.e., people living in an increasingly atomistic, fragmented society, some corporations truly do create some overarching meaning. Moreover, "through their rituals, [such corporations] teach people how to behave, not just in their corridors of power but in the world at large."[5]

And whatever rituals, visions or values have blossomed in the traditions of such corporations *cum* religious communities, the ground from which they have sprouted is the same as that for any other human community, whether religious or otherwise—*a story* of a corporate past arcing toward some future. For those remaining faithful to their storyline, the risk of faith is that the future will be one of blessing rather than of curse, of good fortune and not doom.

Covenantal Loyalty

In *After Virtue*, Alasdair MacIntyre calls attention to the centrality of stories for human life by reminding us that "I can only answer the question 'What am I to do?' if I can answer the prior question 'Of what story...do I find myself a part?' "[6] In other words, larger communal stories frame our individual life stories, thereby framing our identities as well.

Often cast as histories, such communal narratives, by requiring that we look back at significant persons and events in the past, implicitly suggest significant characters and occurrences for us to look for in the future. In short, such stories impart to us *a vision*. That vision shows us a future in which, according to MacIntyre,

> ...certain possibilities beckon us forward and others repel us, some seem already foreclosed and others perhaps inevitable....If the narrative of our [life] is to continue intelligibly...it is always both the case that there are constraints on how the story can continue *and* that within those constraints there are indefinitely many ways it can continue.[7]

Such classical communal stories, therefore, invite their hearers to think of themselves as participants in an embodied narrative quest toward some future goal or end.[8] As a consequence, these same stories will also provide their hearers guidance in what will be "counted as harm and danger and...how success and failure, progress and its opposite, are understood and evaluated."[9] Thus, prominently depicted in these stories will be certain *recurring kinds of performances* or *practices*; also strikingly displayed will be certain *habitual ways of performing those practices* or *virtues*. For those who would embark on the quests recounted in the narrated traditions of story-based communities, practices and virtues are indispensable moral resources because they have the power to

> ...sustain us in the relevant kind of quest for the good by enabling us to overcome the harms, dangers, temptations and distractions which we encounter, and which will furnish us with increasing self-knowledge and increasing knowledge of the good [desired].[10]

Stories, by giving us a vision of communal quests toward some end accompanied by the requisite practices and virtues, thereby give us our "values."[11]

Israel's exodus from Egypt is just such a story.[12] It is a narrative about a quest embarked upon by a community-in-formation toward a common goal—the fulfillment of a promise:

> The Lord said to Abram, "Go forth from your native land and from your father's house to the land that I will show you. I will make of you a great nation, and I will bless you; I will make your name great, and you shall be a blessing. I will bless those who bless you and curse him

who curses you. All the families of the earth shall bless themselves by you." (Gen. 12:1-3)

It is the dynamic of that promise's fulfillment which drives the narrative forward. No matter how many twists and turns the story line may take—a Hebrew baby raised by the daughter of the Hebrews' genocidal enemy, a speech-impeded man called to be spokesman *par excellence*, a forty-year wilderness trek to kill off the generation just rescued—certain outcomes nevertheless are precluded: Israel may no more turn back to Egypt any more than she may worship a golden calf.[13] Instead, an altogether different destiny is envisaged, an entirely different vision summoned up:

> Now then, if you will obey Me faithfully and keep My covenant, you shall be My treasured possession among all the peoples. Indeed, all the earth is Mine, but you shall be to Me a kingdom of priests and a holy nation. (Ex. 19:5-6)

But the narrated keeping of the promise does more than dramatically power the story forward. It calls into existence also a practice and a virtue absolutely essential for the existence of the community of Israel; the practice is *remembering*, the virtue, *faithfulness*. In the Exodus narrative, it is an act of remembering that triggers the chain of events leading to Israel's eventual deliverance:

> The Israelites were groaning under the bondage and cried out; and their cry for help from the bondage rose up to God. God heard their moaning, and God remembered his covenant with Abraham and Isaac and Jacob. (Ex. 2:23-24)

Later, another act of remembering preserves Israel when, although recently delivered from Egyptian servitude and pledged to serve the Lord, she renders him false service instead:

> The Lord spoke to Moses, "Your people...have acted basely. They have been quick to turn aside from the way that I enjoined upon them. They have made themselves a molten calf and bowed low to it....
> "Now, let me be, that my anger may blaze forth against them, and that I may destroy them...."
> But Moses implored the Lord his God, saying, "Let not your anger, Oh Lord, blaze forth against your people....Turn from your blazing

anger, and renounce the plan to punish your people. Remember your servants, Abraham, Isaac, and Jacob, how you swore to them..., 'I will make your offspring as numerous as the stars of heaven, and I will give to your offspring this whole land of which I spoke, to possess forever.' "

And the Lord renounced the punishment he had planned to bring upon his people. (Ex. 32:7-8, 10-14)

For the community of Israel, remembering past promises is indispensable for realizing whatever promise the future may hold.

But remembering the past, like keeping a promise, requires one virtue above all others: faithfulness. In the Hebrew Bible, the word that typically expresses that virtue is *chesed*. The term, appearing in one form or another over two hundred times in Scripture, has at bottom a specific, quasi-technical meaning: "covenantal loyalty."[14] In the Exodus narrative, the paradigmatic exemplar of that virtue is God. Thus, in an act of covenantal renewal following Israel's transgression with the calf, God reveals to Moses his hallmark character trait, i.e., his chief virtue, which enables him to renew the covenant in the first place: "The Lord! A God compassionate and gracious, slow to anger, rich in covenantal loyalty [*chesed*], showing faithfulness [*chesed*] to thousands...." (Ex. 34:6-7) As important, Moses has whatever authority and leadership he possesses precisely because in ways similar to God's, he, too, displays that singular virtue. As depicted in the Exodus narrative, neither God nor Moses is particularly charismatic, or particularly eloquent, or particularly good at "managing" people.[15] And yet, they both excel at steadfastly persevering to realize the ends they seek. Since Israel's continued existence depends on just such steadfast devotion, God and Moses are, not surprisingly, the heroes of the story which Israel tells from generation to generation.

Are there similar stories to be told—and heard—in corporate America?

Corporate "Saints"

For those who hold them, shared values define the fundamental character of their organization...that distinguishes [it] from all others....[Such values] create a special sense of identity..., giving meaning to work as something more than...earning a living....Sometimes managers refer explicitly to...these values in [guiding] sub-ordinates....*New people may be told stories about the company's past that underline the importance of these values to the company.*[16]

As in any corporate *cultus,* General Electric's employees are deeply devoted to its values, and in any recitation of those values, the company's motto stands as the central tenet of its corporate creed: "Progress Is Our Most Important Product." Yet even more fundamental than that corporate article of faith are General Electric's stories about the GE heroes, the GE *saints,* who gave rise to it *by embodying it.*

One of those corporate saints is Thomas Edison, a figure revered not only in GE's pantheon of heroes, but in the larger American society outside GE as well. Virtually every American schoolchild knows the story of Edison conducting experiment after experiment to find the right filament for the electric light. And virtually every GE employee knows the story of Edison's developing the vehicle for simultaneous two-way telegraphic communication: After spending twenty-two consecutive nights testing twenty-three different duplexes, he finally invented one that worked.[17]

Another such GE saint is Charles Steinmetz, a man whose own life coincided with Edison's in many ways. He worked in Edison's lab, which he ran after Edison left.[18] Like Edison, Steinmetz suffered from a physical disability.[19] Like Edison, Steinmetz played a large part in GE's growth as a company; he "brought alternating current into electrical systems of the world."[20] And, like Edison, stories about his work at GE germinated values which, along with their corporate exemplar, are revered to this day—as the following episode reported by one of the authors of *Corporate Cultures* makes clear:

> We drove by the General Electric Research Lab where—in an earlier era and building—Charles Steinmetz had conducted his experiments. The driver of the car motioned to the building and said, "Sometimes I get the feeling I can still see the lights on in there and Steinmetz working away." For the driver, and for other employees of GE *who never knew Steinmetz,* he still was a strong influence....[21]

Not for nothing is *inventing GE's cardinal practice*[22] while *persistence*[23] is *its cardinal virtue.*

But Steinmetz plays a saintly role in GE's lore in another way. He is responsible for creating the vision that stands at the heart of the company's story-based self-understanding as a community of inventive engineers and scientists with *close personal ties* to one another:

Whenever young engineers joined GE, Steinmetz would invite them home for the weekend in order to learn, sincerely and without political intent, what kind of people they were. Once he adopted one of GE's leading engineers as his own son—and the man's whole family. They all moved into Steinmetz's house and lived with him for twenty years.[24]

With this bit of hagiography as background, General Electric nurtures a corporate cult which emulates the saintliness of Steinmetz through fostering supportiveness, loyalty and respect among peer-group members.

Thus, like vibrant religious communities, some corporations have stories in which a venerated past bears promise for the future. In fact, many writers have suggested that companies displaying high financial performance and potential are precisely those with powerful narrative traditions.[25]

But is this account of the implications of story-based values for corporations, like some medieval morality play, a story too good to be true?

Excellent or Victorious?

MacIntyre would almost certainly answer, "Yes." For him, while classical societies tended to reflect a single unified—and unifying—core narrative, modern culture reflects many different story fragments, thereby shattering our moral vision as well. Corporate life, for its part, fragments the moral life even more:

Within any one large formal organization not only variety, but incoherence is to be found [since] corporate structures fragment consciousness and more especially moral consciousness.[26]

Corporate existence...presupposes a separation of spheres of existence, a moral distancing of each social role from each of the others.[27]

In MacIntyre's view, corporate life splits the moral life into (at least) two distinct and incompatible realms—that of the individual corporate employee governed by utilitarian considerations and that of the family member or citizen whose moral considerations are anything but utilitarian.[28] Consequently, for MacIntyre, the corporation, far from providing the closest thing our society has to community, comes close to being the institutional embodiment of a modern, individualistic ethos—the very antithesis of any genuine notion of community.

And yet, MacIntyre may well have gotten his labels reversed. For it may well be that in contemporary U.S. society, the corporation in its basic structure and daily operation is the last bastion of any truly functioning community while, for their parts, modern politics and the modern family run on little more than fleeting individual preferences and fickle personal desires.[29] By contrast, as MacIntyre himself admits, corporate

> organization [must] be conceived in terms of roles and not of persons. Any role, any position, will be filled from time to time by different persons....Correspondence for example is conducted with this or that office of the organization and not—except accidentally—with individuals. Hence the formal character of bureaucratic correspondence; hence the importance of files. Each file has a history [i.e., *a narrative*] which outlives that of the individuals who contribute to it.[30]

Indeed, many observers have taken note of the role that so-called "excellent companies" play in creating an entire reality for those working in them; even more than that, for many corporate employees, the reality thus created catches them up in something transcendent, even bordering on the religious. As Tom Peters has remarked in his best-selling book, *In Search of Excellence*:

> By offering *meaning* as well as money, [the excellent companies] give their employees a *mission* as well as a sense of feeling great. Every man becomes a pioneer, an experimenter, a leader. The institution provides *guiding belief* and creates a sense of excitement, *a sense of being part* of the best....[31]

In fact, at a time when the general culture provides little or no stability regarding values, corporations may play an especially crucial role by providing "structure and standards and a value system in which to operate."[32] In just that way, "corporations may be among the last institutions in America that can effectively take on the role of shaping values."[33]

Nevertheless, MacIntyre might still object that, within the corporation, values are not shaped but shattered as mixed signals are sent regarding them such that the same moral chaos pervades the workplace as any other place in contemporary American society:

> Unfortunately the very same quality is often presented in one guise as a virtue, in another as a vice. The same executive is characteristically required to be meticulous in adhering to routines...*and* to show initiative....Especially perhaps among upwardly mobile middle management, contemporaries in the organization are presented at one and the same time as those *with* whom he or she is expected to cooperate and *against* whom he or she is expected to complete.[34]

Such conflicting imperatives, however, need not *necessarily* indicate moral anarchy. On the contrary, their conflict may arise in the first place precisely because they both spring from a moral outlook more fundamentally shared than shattered. In *Antigone*, for instance, the protagonist is faced with the dilemma of two apparently incommensurate moral claims—those calling her to honor her familial and religious obligations to bury her dead brother versus those calling her to keep her political obligations to deny burial to a traitor to the state. As a consequence, no matter how Antigone acts, her act can and will appear at one and the same time both a display of virtue—loyalty—and of vice—betrayal. Yet we must not miss the fact that this conflict between moral obligations in *Antigone* grows out of a unified, coherent moral vision in which life, its values, and its goods are understood principally in terms of concrete relationships, roles and duties rather than abstract principles, rights and "oughts."[35]

Similarly, the underlying tension between cooperation and competition in corporate life may stem from a deeper shared commitment to a common goal or good. We can think, for example, of a high school basketball team in which competition between team members exists side-by-side with cooperation among them for the sake of realizing a common purpose. In the context of practice, for instance, team skills such as the fast break and the zone defense—which demand cooperation among the team's members—coexist with competition between individuals to increase their respective amounts of playing time or crack the starting lineup. What must not be overlooked is that *both* cooperation *and* competition must be employed if the team itself is to achieve excellence and especially the excellence needed to be a champion prevailing over all opponents. And so, too, if a company wants to achieve preeminence over other companies, its members must learn cooperation as well as competition.

But MacIntyre, undaunted, still might object that where achievement of excellence is equated with achievement of victory, any notion of virtue is summarily defeated—along with any claims to moral seriousness made on behalf of the corporation. For excellence and victory, though closely related, are nevertheless distinct concepts: after all, it is possible *to be excellent yet lose.* To see the difference between being excellent and being victorious, just look, says MacIntyre, at "the Spartan sacrifice at Thermopylae."[36]

But witness, too, the fact that even the excellent high school basketball team can lose, through poor officiating costing it a crucial free-throw opportunity or poor grades costing it the services of its star. And witness also the fact that even a corporation may choose to court loss(es) to maintain certain standards of excellence: just witness the case of Johnson & Johnson during the Tylenol scare.

In the fall of 1982, seven people died when they swallowed Extra-Strength Tylenol capsules laced with cyanide. At the time, Tylenol was the top-selling health and beauty aid product in the U.S.[37] Its corporate parent, Johnson & Johnson, had built the company reputation on trust and responsibility going back to its founding as an innovator in supplying sterile surgical dressings. Now, J&J was faced with the very real possibility that if it acted in a trustworthy and responsible fashion, it might lose not only its premier product in the marketplace but a significant slice of its total corporate revenues.

Nevertheless, within the first few days following the poisonings, the company, under the leadership of its chairman, James Burke, withdrew virtually its whole Tylenol line from market shelves and ceased all Tylenol advertising. Within a week, J&J stock had dropped about 20 percent, amounting to a paper loss of $2 billion. But said Burke, "It's important that we demonstrate that we've taken every single step possible to protect the public...."[38] Hardly, it would seem, the words of someone blind to the difference between excellence and winning.

As events wore on, Burke stayed the course he had set. The consensus of his advertising consultants was that the Tylenol name was dead, and many such as media maven Jerry Della Femina were adamant that the Tylenol name had to be changed before the product could be reintroduced. But Burke—and J&J—held firm. Remarked Wayne Nelson, J&J Company group chairman, "It would almost be an admission of guilt...to walk away from that name."[39]   Echoing Nelson's remarks, Burke said on the *Donahue* show:

> It seems to me that there is a certain not playing it straight with the consumers on that one. If you are going to sell Tylenol, to sell it under a name other than its own name is kind of asking you to change your name after you've had a serious disease....[40]

Throughout the whole affair, Burke and J&J stuck to their conviction that informing and protecting the nation would result eventually in "an eminently fair decision about the future of Tylenol."[41]   In the end, the company saw its *commitment to excellence* in reliably providing health care *vindicated.* Within a year of the crisis, Tylenol had regained over 90 percent of the market it had enjoyed prior to the tragedies.[42] And in the 1990 *Fortune* magazine polling for America's most admired companies, J&J won top honors for its commitment to community and environmental responsibility.[43]

Even so, however, MacIntyre might once more mount a protest: The corporate practices of even a company like J&J have no real moral power or depth to them because none of the goods pursued through those practices are *internal* to them.   That is, in the course of pursuing the standards of excellence appropriate to and definitive of J&J's business activities, no good intrinsically related to such activities is realized, nor, for that matter, is any human power to achieve excellence or any human conception of the good involved systematically extended.[44] At best, only certain external or contingent goods are realized, such as money or power.

But the matter is not so easily settled. If we recall for a moment the key practice at General Electric—inventing—we discover that the chief good internal to the practice is the very one named in the company's motto: progress. And as GE's corporate story makes clear, progress is a good which would be difficult, if not impossible, to achieve without invention and without the virtue necessary to sustain that practice, namely, persistence. As for J&J, it is a company at whose heart stands a *credo*, a corporate catechism of convictions concerning its responsibilities to its customers, its employees, its community and its shareholders— in just that order. To provide products and services in pursuit of health— an internal good if ever there was one—J&J must cultivate exactly those virtues it demonstrated during the Tylenol crisis: trustworthiness, practical wisdom, and courage.[45]

MacIntyre has pointed out that "in the ancient and medieval worlds the creation and sustaining of human communities—of households, cities, and nations—is generally taken to be a practice....[46] And so, too, ought we to take the creation and sustaining of certain corporate communities in the modern world. Hence, all moral misgivings regarding the corporation in its modern form would seem to be unwarranted.

Or are they? Before answering, we would be wise to hear the whole story of the rise of the modern American corporation.

Incorporation

Are the vultures still out there? — Former Drexel staffer, sneering at reporters as she walked out the door following the firm's announcement of bankruptcy.

Vultures? Look who's talking. — Security guard (*Time*, 2/26/90).

Earlier, we spoke of monastic communities as being among the first corporations, as being bodies of persons joined to pursue a common enterprise.[47] Such bodies, however, were not interested in benefitting only their own members; they aimed at benefitting those outside them as well. As Trachtenberg and Foner have reminded us, "It was assumed, as it is still in nonprofit corporations, that the incorporated body earned its charter by serving the public good."[48] Similarly, the authors of *Habits of the Heart* have pointed out that "incorporation [was] a concession of public authority to a private group *in return* for service to the public good...."[49] Again, from the times of the earliest monastic orders, such corporate communities sought to contribute to the common good beyond the monastery walls. For example, "because of the paramount obligations of charity toward one's fellow man, [St. Basil] established [his monasteries] in towns instead of in desert wastes," while his forerunner, Pachomius, generated his *Koinonia* or monastic community out of a broader commitment to "the service of humankind."[50]

Clearly, such corporate models presupposed a model of society in which it made sense to speak of "the common good." But as American society became more and more industrialized following the Civil War, notions of the common good became less and less coherent. The bonds among Americans, both political and economic, grew increasingly attenuated. Whereas in the earlier life of the Republic the dominant social metaphor was the town meeting where all joined in an effort to reach consensus to pursue a common good, the regnant image after the Civil War was the marketplace where each pursued his or her own good. At best indifferent to and at worst hostile to the goods pursued by others, each was bound to those others only by a few thin procedures meant to ensure that competition was—at least minimally—"fair."

Such was the social climate that spawned the modern business corporation. As Lawrence Friedman has noted, in the late nineteenth century "the overriding need was for an efficient, trouble-free device to aggregate capital and manage it in business, with limited liability and transferable shares."[51] And here, the idea of "limited liability" is crucial, for the novel legal fiction giving the corporation the status of a "person" meshed perfectly with the social fabric of the times. In an age celebrating *laissez-faire* competition among rugged individuals, concocting a "super-individual" to join the fray was a master stroke. Better still, if the fray proved to be too hot and the adversaries too strong, then even though the corporation's legal person might be bested, its human persons, still shielded by the doctrine of limited liability, could withdraw unscathed with their own resources intact. As a result, incorporation, which once had been a rare privilege granted only by special charter for the sake of the common good, became an ever-present right routinely available by application to any private enterprise.[52]

Thus, the creation stories of many U.S. corporations such as Standard Oil and Ford are but retellings of a larger American story, the story of how that newly created corporate person, often through the enterprise and grit of its founder, overcame all obstacles—including other corporate persons in the form of adversarial competitors—while remaining oblivious to any good but its own.

Corporate Responsibility

Accordingly, in a society where the notion of a common good has long since died, to find corporations acting without any regard for such a good is hardly surprising. Why, for instance, should anyone be surprised to find R.J. Reynolds attempting to regain lost cigarette sales by targeting its advertising for new brands at blacks and young women? In the fragmented, atomistic America of the late twentieth century, the burden of making a *coherent* moral argument is heavier for RJR's critics than it is for the company.

In its earlier days, of course, the company at least displayed commitment to those who fell within the orbit of its own corporate community. It provided adequate day care for workers' children, it offered RJR stock as well as liberal loans to its employees, and it gave generous gifts to its hometown of Winston-Salem. And yet, as it continued to flourish in a culture which increasingly lost sight of any *shared* good, RJR's commitments to share even with those in its own purview grew gradually weaker. Thus, in connection with the RJR Nabisco takeover, at least 5,100 employees eventually were thrown out of work while the company virtually pulled out of Winston-Salem. In the leveraged buyout's aftermath, former RJR employees in Winston-Salem were besieged by brokers and buyers offering to buy their now highly valuable stock. In response, the townspeople asked incredulously, "You want to buy *stock*?" Explained Nabley Armfield, a local stockbroker, "You have to understand. Reynolds wasn't a stock, it was a *religion*."[53]

But to the extent that U.S. culture makes corporations like RJR Nabisco unsurprising, to just that extent, the corporate culture of a company like Johnson & Johnson is truly astonishing for binding the company to some larger, shared notion of the good. Like some religious order formed in another time and place, the Johnson & Johnson community lives by a *credo*:

> We are responsible to the communities in which we live and work and to the world community as well. We must be good citizens—support good works and charities and bear our fair share of taxes. We must encourage civic improvements and better health and education. We must maintain in good order the property we are privileged to use, protecting the environment and natural resources.

For J&J, these words are not some part of a dead doxology intoned as an ancient, fossilized rite. Instead, it is a living text which is revised periodically to keep J&J's corporate vision alive and vital. Hence, looking back on the "Tylenol nightmare" in which "literally dozens of people [had] to make hundreds of decisions in painfully short periods of time," James Burke could say with wholehearted conviction, "All of us...truly believe that the guidance of the *credo* played *the* most important role in our decision-making."[54]

Nor are J&J and Burke alone in witnessing to a corporate life with striking similarities to certain aspects of religious life; they are joined by Herman Miller, Inc., and its chairman, Max De Pree. In the previously mentioned *Fortune* listing of the nation's most admired companies, Herman Miller ranked ninth overall while taking sixth place for management excellence. In a newspaper interview, De Pree expressed the following convictions about corporate life:

[A reason for America's lack of leaders] is that people have felt it was OK to put themselves ahead of the common good.

[Leadership is not a question] of techniques...but of what is in the heart.

Corporations can and should have a redemptive purpose....[55]

De Pree's convictions about the corporation are nothing if not religious—especially this one: "Being faithful to a set of beliefs is more important than being successful."[56]

That claim, perhaps more than any other, raises the question as to whether some forms of corporate life can genuinely be considered as instances of the religious life. Would any corporation be willing to remain faithful to its values *even unto death*? If doing good and doing well do not necessarily go hand in hand, then corporations may need to weigh carefully the stories they live out: Not all of them may have happy endings.

Stories and Values

Stories and values are not only sources of corporate performance; at one level, they are also constraints against it:

Although [shared values] provide a source of clear common understanding in a business, they also constitute a constraint. When a company with strongly held values finds that [it has] lost marketplace or economic relevance, it generally has great difficulty adjusting successfully.[57]

A storied past thus not only informs us but, displaying a vision to guide our present and future, also *forms us* in the way we envisage our world and our options for acting in it. Not for nothing do some 70 percent of corporate mergers fail as companies find themselves unable to merge their separate—and often incompatible—story lines into a new ongoing narrative.[58] In such circumstances, corporate stories may spell death instead of life.

In the last analysis, the most basic test of any story, whether corporate, religious or some other, is the kind of life that it produces and, even more fundamentally, whether it produces any life at all; stories die when their communal embodiments do—which is only fitting justice. Hence, without Zeus worshippers, what are the stories of Zeus *but* stories?

Granted, it may take a relatively long time for a community and its culture to see whether the story they have been living out may actually be leading to their demise. Corporate cultures, however, may come by such knowledge more quickly due to the rapid feedback the marketplace provides. That feedback may carry with it possible correctives to prevent the company's story from having yet reached its final chapter. Thus, at the height of the Tylenol crisis, Burke told a press conference:

> We consider it a moral imperative, as well as good business, to restore Tylenol to its preeminent position in the marketplace. It is ironic that the job of rebuilding Tylenol is made more difficult because we all...did our job of informing and protecting the nation so efficiently. In the final analysis, we believe that the American consumer...will make an eminently fair decision about the future of Tylenol.[59]

Burke had faith that J&J's willingness to continue to live out its traditional story line would be matched by the market's willingness to let the company continue to live. J&J's willingness to act on that article of faith was what made its *credo credible*.

Consequently, to dismiss business ethics such as J&J's as "*merely utilitarian*" is unwarranted. When executives like Burke "bet the company," they take nothing more nor less than a risk of faith. In that regard, faith such as theirs may well resemble that of some religious communities during times of persecution, as reflected, for example, by this teaching from Jewish tradition:

> At a time of persecution when...decrees are issued against Israel aimed at abolishing their religious practice..., then let [a Jew] suffer death and not breach even one of...the commandments.[60]

Jewish tradition here makes sense precisely to the extent that there *is* a truly steadfast King of Kings to come to Israel's rescue before the life of the last Jewish man or woman is sacrificed. If Jews were to act on this teaching and the whole Jewish people subsequently were to perish, then, although the teaching may have been foolish, it will most assuredly *not* have been utilitarian. And the same could have been said about the *credo*'s teaching had J&J perished during the Tylenol crisis.

Yet, for all the virtues and all the faith that a company like Johnson & Johnson has shown, the virtues and the faith displayed, although in certain key ways religious, are in no way *biblical.*[61] For neither their "structurings of reality" nor their "ultimate concerns" are unified finally with the One who, according to the Bible's story, has made all of life corporate by having created all of it, sustained all of it and, for Christians at least, redeemed all of it. In contrast, for those communities formed by even the most exemplary of modern corporations, the horizons of their moral vision extend no farther than the boundaries of their market. By comparison, a community whose vision has been expanded by the lenses provided by biblical narrative may yet be able to see *the whole of creation as one corpus*, with the blessing of life offered as a common good above any individual partial goods.

Yet modern corporations tussling in the marketplace have no goods to offer but partial—and often conflicting—ones. In the pursuit of such limited goods, companies may ask for unlimited commitment from their employees; indeed, it may be precisely the most conscientious companies which ask for the most commitment—whether an Edison-like dedication to round-the-clock inventing or a *credo*-like fidelity to put one's customers above all else. And yet, such commitment, even in the best of contemporary corporate communities and even with all the attendant piety, still falls short of having singleminded, wholehearted devotion to God. Hence, whatever practices such commitment may engender, those whose corporate vision has been shaped by biblical narrative—Jews, Christians, Muslims—may recognize such practices by another name: idolatry.

At present, such vision may be particularly difficult to attain, not merely because the biblical notion of idolatry seems so hopelessly anachronistic but, more fundamentally, because the very corporations engaged in idol worship appear in many other ways to be so virtuous, so admirable, so noble. But, after all, that is the way it is with *noble pagans*. For them, religious practice does not consist of child sacrifice nor do their values find expression in drunken orgies. Instead, virtue for such noble ones as these lies in paying due homage to the many gods, the many powers, and the many roles at work in the *agora* and the forum.

Thus, as America's corporate communities move into the first century of the next millennium, they may carry with them the religious values of the first century of the first millennium. Those values, of course, derive from a story that in fundamental ways differs from any narrative called "biblical." Consequently, no matter the millennium, no matter the community, the bottom line issue remains the same: In which story and in which values ought we to invest our lives?[62]

Notes

1. Robert A. Irvin and Edward G. Michaels, III, "Core Skills: Doing the Right Things Right," *The McKinsey Quarterly*, 25, Summer 1989, p. 10.

2. *Ibid.*, p. 8.

3. Warren Bennis and Burt Nanus, *Leaders* (New York: Harper & Row, 1985), p. 83.

4. Alan Trachtenberg and Eric Foner, *The Incorporation of America: Culture and Society in the Gilded Age* (New York: Hill and Wang, 1982), p. 5; emphasis added.
As for St. Benedict, his Rule gives "directions for the formation, government, and administration of a monastery and for the spiritual and daily life of its monks....The Rule provides for an autonomous, self-contained community (66)....The monastery of the Rule is a microcosm containing inmates of every age and condition...." (B. Colgrave, "Benedictine Rule," *New Catholic Encyclopedia*).

5. Terrence E. Deal and Allen A. Kennedy, *Corporate Cultures* (Reading, MA: Addison-Wesley Publishing Co., Inc., 1982), p. 83. Though subtitled *The Rites and Rituals of Corporate Life*, the book contains precious little that approaches corporate life from the vantage point of religious life or, for that matter, religious studies. Instead, the volume and its bibliography are top-heavy with standard fare of business organization.
Let me be clear here. My point here is *not* that corporate life can be understood *only* from the perspective of religion; obviously, it can be analyzed from other standpoints as well, e.g., economics, sociology, social psychology and the like. However, I am suggesting that various forms of religious life may offer rather fruitful ways for thinking about certain instances of corporate life, together with their visions and their values. In that respect, my primary task in this essay is more descriptive than prescriptive.

6. Alasdair MacIntyre, *After Virtue* (Notre Dame, IN: University of Notre Dame Press, 1981), p. 201.

7. *Ibid.*, pp. 200-201.

8. *Ibid.*, p. 203.

9. *Ibid.*, p. 135.

10. *Ibid.*, p. 204.

11. I have set the word *values* in quotes to call attention to the fact that for ethics, that notion reflects a particularly modern understanding—namely, that in the last analysis, there are no moral goods or standards apart from individual preferences, desires and wants. For powerful critiques of this position, cf. MacIntyre, Chapter Two, "The Nature of Moral Disagreement Today and the Claims of Emotivism," and Allan Bloom, *The Closing of the American Mind* (New York: Simon & Schuster, 1987), pp. 60-61.
The fact that American business as a whole tends to use "values" as synonymous for—and to the virtual exclusion of other terms such as "ethics," "goods" and "standards" indicates that even for the corporation, an institution whose pre-modern motifs can still be heard, the trope of modernity is nevertheless inescapable.

12. See my *Jews and Christians, Getting Our Stories Straight* (Nashville: Abingdon, 1985).

13. Cf., e.g., Ex. 16:3, 17:3 and 32:25-35.

14. See Nelson Glueck, *[Ch]esed in the Bible,* trans. A. Gottschalk (Cincinnati: Hebrew Union College Press, 1967). Even if one prefers a less technical rendering of *chesed,* such as, for instance, the RSV's "steadfast love," the term's basic thrust remains the same: faithful devotion.

15. See MacIntyre's description on p. 29 of the manager and therapist as embodying quintessentially modern roles which enable them to manipulate people to achieve certain ends, without regard for any moral concerns about such manipulation or such ends.

16. Julien R. Phillips and Allen A. Kennedy, "Shaping and Managing Shared Values," *McKinsey Staff Paper,* December 1980, p.4; emphasis added.

17. *Ibid.*, p. 11.

18. Deal and Kennedy, p. 45.

19. Steinmetz was crippled while Edison, having had his ears "boxed" as a child, suffered from a serious hearing loss.

20. Deal and Kennedy, p. 8.

21. *Ibid.*, p. 47.

22. For a discussion of the relationship between practices and goods, see MacIntyre, p. 175, and my discussion below on pp. 18-19.

23. In fact, much of the current literature on leadership points to persistence as being the outstanding character trait—that is, virtue—of those considered leaders. See, e.g., Deal and Kennedy, p. 46; Bennis and Nanus, pp. 45, 47,

187-88; Phillips and Kennedy, pp. 18, 19; and Nigel Williams, "Managing Values on Wall Street," keynote speech to the Securities Industry Association Conference, October 29, 1987, p. 9.

Perhaps a necessary—though not sufficient—condition for any leader is a single-minded willingness to act out a vision and live out a story. Thomas Peters, referring to the work of Bennis and Nanus, points out that leaders have clear visions, which are "lived with almost frightening consistency...." *(Thriving on Chaos: Handbook for a Management Revolution* [New York: Perennial Library, 1987], p. 631). That observation may help to remind us that corporate communities, particularly in their early days, are often like religious cults—that is, they are tightly organized around a central person: *the cult figure.* If that person is a cult figure like Jesus of Nazareth, well and good; if, however, that person is a cult figure like Jim Jones....

24. Deal and Kennedy, p. 45.

25. *Ibid.*, pp. 7, 30. Cf. also Williams, p. 5; Phillips and Kennedy, pp. 2, 12; and Alan Wilkins, "Organizational Stories as an Expression of Management Philosophy," Ph.D. dissertation, Stanford University, 1978.

26. Alasdair MacIntyre, "Corporate Modernity and Moral Judgment: Are They Mutually Exclusive?" in *Ethics and Problems of the 21st Century*, eds. K.E. Goodpaster and K.M. Sayre (Notre Dame, IN: University of Notre Dame Press, 1979), p. 122.

27. *Ibid.*, p. 126.

28. *Ibid.*, pp. 126-27.

29. Regarding contemporary politics, MacIntyre himself has written, "Modern politics is civil war carried on by other means" *(After Virtue*, p. 236). As for the modern family, see Robert N. Bellah, Richard Madsen, William Sullivan, Ann Swidler and Steven M. Tipton, "Love and Marriage," Chapter Four, *Habits of the Heart: Individualism and Commitment in American Life* (New York: Harper & Row, 1985). See also Christopher Lasch's *Haven in a Heartless World: The Family Besieged* (New York: Basic Books, 1977); for many Americans, the family might be likened to an emotional gas station, where they drop by to tank up on affection before pulling out into social traffic once more.

30. MacIntyre, "Corporate Modernity and Moral Judgment," p. 124.

31. Thomas J. Peters and Robert H. Waterman, Jr., *In Search of Excellence: Lessons from America's Best-Run Companies* (New York: Warner Books, 1982), p. 323; emphasis added.

32. Deal and Kennedy, p. 16.

33. *Ibid.*

34. MacIntyre, "Corporate Modernity and Moral Judgment," p. 123.

35. Cf. Alasdair MacIntyre, *Against the Self-Images of the Age* (New York: Schocken Books, 1971), pp. 123-24, 168-69.

36. Alasdair MacIntyre, *Whose Justice? Which Rationality* (Notre Dame, IN: University of Notre Dame Press, 1988), pp. 27-28.

37. Thomas J.C. Raymond with Elisabeth Ament Lipton, "Tylenol," *Harvard Business School Case* (Boston: President and Fellows of Harvard College, 1984), p. 1.

38. *Ibid.*, pp. 2-3.

39. *Ibid.*, p. 4.

40. *Ibid.*, p. 11.

41. *Ibid.*, p. 10.

42. James E. Burke, "The Leverage of Goodwill," speech to the Advertising Council, November 16, 1983, p. 4.

43. "Leadership of the Most Admired," *Fortune*, January 29, 1990, p. 50.

44. MacIntyre, *After Virtue*, p. 175.

45. Cf. Jeffrey Stout, *Ethics After Babel* (Boston: Beacon, 1988), p. 269. Speaking of medical practice, Richard Vance insightfully has pointed out that *contra* Stout (and thus MacIntyre as well), there is not so wide or clear a gap between internal and external goods as we have been led to believe:

> Yet medicine as a craft has always, even in Hippocratic times, considered remuneration to be closely connected to the quality of care. Money and prestige are not, of course, direct goals of medical practice, but they are not merely external attachments either. One need not be a cynic...to note that financial issues are more complexly related to medical practice than Stout's analysis admits ("We Are All Pragmatists Now: The Limits of Modern Medical Ethics in American Medical Education" [unpublished paper, 1989], p. 16).

Vance's observation concerning medical practice obviously has implications for other kinds of practices as well.

46. MacIntyre, *After Virtue*, p. 175.

47. *Ibid.*, p. 2.

48. Trachtenberg and Foner, pp. 5-6.

49. Bellah, et al., p. 290.

50. St. Basil, *Ascetical Works*, trans. Sr. Monica M. Wagner, C.S.C. (New York: Fathers of the Church, Inc., 1950), p. xi; Armand Veilleux, trans. and intro., *The Life of Saint Pachomius and His Disciples*, foreword by Adalbert de Vogué, vol. 1, Cistercian Studies Series, no. 45 (Kalamazoo, MI: Cistercian Publications, Inc., 1980), p. xvii.

51. Lawrence M. Friedman, *A History of American Law*, 2nd ed. (New York: Simon & Schuster, 1985), p. 201.

52. Trachtenberg and Foner, p. 6.

53. Bryan Burrough and John Helyar, *Barbarians at the Gate: The Fall of RJR Nabisco* (New York: Harper & Row, 1990), pp. 45, 49, 91, 511; emphasis added.

54. Burke, pp. 3-4.
55. *Atlanta Journal Constitution*, December 11, 1989, sec. B, p. 6.
56. *Ibid.*
57. Phillips and Kennedy, p. 5.
58. Peters and Waterman, Jr., pp. 292-93, and McKinsey & Co. research.
59. Raymond with Lipton, p. 10.
60. Maimonides, Mishneh Torah, Hilchot Yesodei HaTorah, 5:3.
61. A failure to see this difference can result in the kind of business apologia written by Michael Novak; cf. his *Toward a Theology of the Corporation* (Washington, D.C.: American Enterprise Institute, 1981), and *The Spirit of Democratic Capitalism* (New York: Simon and Schuster, 1982).
62. I am especially indebted to Richard Vance, James McClendon and Thee Smith for helping me clarify my thinking in this last section of the paper. I want to thank them also for their overall care and responsiveness in replying to an earlier draft of this essay.

Three

Narrative Theology and Business Ethics: Story-Based Management of Values

Charles S. McCoy

In the *Republic* (359d-360d) Plato tells the story of Gyges the Lydian:

> ...a shepherd in the service of the ruler at that time of Lydia, and that after a great deluge of rain and an earthquake the ground opened and a chasm appeared in the place where he was pasturing, and they say that he saw and wondered and went down into the chasm. And the story goes that he beheld other marvels there and a hollow bronze horse with little doors, and that he peeped in and saw a corpse within, as it seemed, of more than mortal stature, and that there was nothing else but a gold ring on its hand, which he took off, and so went forth. And when the shepherds held their customary assembly to make their monthly report to the king about the flocks, he also attended, wearing the ring. So as he sat there it chanced that he turned the collet of the ring toward himself, toward the inner part of his hand, and when this took place they say that he became invisible to those who sat by him and they spoke of him as absent, and that he was amazed, and again fumbling with the ring turned the collet outward and so became visible. On noting this he experimented with the ring to see if it possessed this virtue, and he found the result to be that when he turned the collet inward he became invisible, and when outward, visible, and becoming aware of this, he immediately managed things so that he became one of the messengers who went up to the king, and on coming there he seduced the king's wife and with her aid set upon the king and slew him and possessed his kingdom.
>
> If now there should be two such rings, and the just man should put on one and the unjust the other, no one could be found, it would seem, of such adamantine temper as to persevere in justice and endure to refrain his hands from the possessions of others and not touch them, though he might with impunity take what he wished even from the

market place, and enter into houses and lie with whom he pleased, and slay and loose from bonds whomsoever he would, and in all other things conduct himself among mankind as the equal of a god. And in so acting he would do no differently from the other man but both would pursue the same course. And yet this is a great proof, one might argue, that no one is just of his own will but only from constraint, in the belief that justice is not his personal good, inasmuch as every man, when he supposes himself to have the power to do wrong, does wrong. For that there is far more profit for him personally in injustice than in justice is what every man believes, and believes truly, as the proponent of this theory will maintain. For if anyone who had got such a license within his grasp should refuse to do any wrong or lay his hands on others' possessions, he would be regarded as most pitiable and a great fool by all who took note of it, though they would praise him before one another's faces, deceiving one another because of their fear of suffering injustice.[1]

As this story illustrates, Plato's *Dialogues* are, along with the Bible, a rich resource in the Western tradition for linking narrative to theology and ethics. "The Ring of Gyges" suggests several elements central to Plato's perspective on religion and ethics. First, the story makes it clear that human nature is neither unambiguously good nor evil. Even the unjust must give attention to the standards of behavior set by society, standards they could ignore if they were invisible. And even the most just of humans would have difficulty resisting evil if they could act with impunity because of their invisibility. Second, justice has a reality for Plato, different from the reality of stones and bodies, but having a place in the nature of things. It is highly dubious to speak of the fragility of goodness in a world in which the form of the good is basic. Third, the story of Gyges makes it clear that virtue among humans must be regarded as emerging in societal interaction rather than as something inherent in individuals and practiced in society. The ring that makes Gyges invisible lowers drastically the tendency toward acting justly, while visibility imposes an accountability that makes just action more likely.

The stories of David, Bathsheba and Uriah, culminating with Nathan's dramatic pronouncement, "Thou art the man!" (II Samuel 11:1-12:25) and of Jesus's calling Zacchaeus down from a tree and into a life a greater justice and salvation (Luke 19:1-10) contain perspectives on human nature and morals in ways different from, but parallel to, Plato's many stories. In the Bible, narrative is one of the most important ways, perhaps the basic way, that God, the world, humanity, and the interaction among them is expressed and communicated.

Emerging from the biblical context of historical recital and parable, the Christian movement developed with its central convictions embodied in story, stories of the Hebraic past and the story of Jesus. The shift from the story paradigm to the rational paradigm, or Constantinian paradigm, is described in my book:

> ...shaping the new theological paradigm that emerged in the early centuries of the Christian movement is the institutional church as it became a powerful societal agency in the era after the conversion of Constantine. In this time, stable doctrine was needed. Rather than stories told by believers, theology gradually became the official dogmas defined by church councils and upheld by politically potent ecclesiastical organizations. Faith as right doctrine—orthodoxy became more important than faith as trust and loyalty or as doing the will of God—orthopraxis. In the Constantinian era, theology became organizationally rationalized just as it became philosophically rationalized.[2]

This paradigm also has been dealt with more extensively in Hans Frei's *The Eclipse of Biblical Narrative.*[3] For ethics, the extreme examples of rationalistic methodology were achieved perhaps in the 1960s. In the 1970s and 1980s the grip of rationalism had been weakening, the Constantinian paradigm was cracking, the importance of story in human community was being rediscovered.

Into the Rational Wasteland

Ethics in general and business ethics in particular has been weakened and eviscerated by the tendencies in recent decades to adopt rationalistic, individualistic models of ethics and to abandon its rootage in story, history and narrative theology. One of the most pervasive methods in philosophy for these models has been linguistic analysis.

Mary Warnock, summarizing her views of *Ethics Since 1900,* has this to say of the analysis of language in ethics:

> One of the consequences of treating ethics as the analysis of language is, as I have suggested earlier, that it leads to the increasing triviality of the subject. This is not a general criticism of linguistic analysis, but only of this method applied to ethics. In ethics, alone among the branches of philosophical study, the subject matter is not so much the

categories which we use to describe or to learn about the world, as our own impact upon the world, our relation to other people and our attitude to our situation and our life. We do need to categorize and to describe, even in the sphere of morals, but we should still exist as moral agents even if we seldom did so; and therefore the subject matter of ethics would still exist....

One aspect of this trivializing of the subject is the refusal of moral philosophers in England to commit themselves to any moral opinions.[4]

One might draw the conclusion, with good reason, that ethicists in the United States, once they had learned from Warnock how to trivialize their subject, set out immediately to do so. It appears to many observers that they succeeded and, indeed, seemed headed on a path of self-destruction.

A professor at a leading business school reported that the faculty became interested in having ethics included in the curriculum, so a philosophical ethicist was invited to address the school. His lecture on Kant was, according to this report, so obscure as to be unintelligible to most of the faculty and students and totally irrelevant for business to those who did understand it. The result, unhappily, was a rejection of the proposal to begin teaching business ethics.

The excursion into the wasteland of rational and linguistic analysis has not been abandoned, but questions about its adequacy to deal with actual situations have been raised with increasing seriousness, and the long march out of the desert has begun. The recovery of human story and narrative theology has been of great help in understanding again the wholeness of experience, in which reason and language play important but not decisive roles.

Resources for Story-Based Ethics

In *The Meaning of Revelation*, perhaps the most important work in theology and ethics published in this century, H. Richard Niebuhr reminds us of a central insight from Alfred North Whitehead as to the core of religious traditions. Whitehead wrote: "Religions commit suicide when they find their inspiration in dogmas. The inspiration of religion lies in the history of religion." I would extend Whitehead's view and say: Ethics commits suicide when it seeks its inspiration in dogma and rationalism; the inspiration of ethics lies in story and history.

In line with the quote from Whitehead, Niebuhr writes as follows in the section of *The Meaning of Revelation* entitled "The Story of Our Life":

> We do well to remind ourselves that the Christian community has usually—and particularly in times of its greatest vigor—used an historical method. Apparently it felt that to speak in confessional terms about the events that had happened to it in its history was not a burdensome necessity but rather an advantage and that the acceptance of an historical point of view was not confining but liberating. The preaching of the early Christian church was not an argument for the existence of God nor an admonition to follow the dictates of some common human conscience, unhistorical and super-social in character. It was primarily a simple recital of the great events connected with the historical appearance of Jesus Christ and a confession of what had happened to the commmunity of disciples. Whatever it was that the church meant to say, whatever was revealed or manifested to it could be indicated only in connection with an historical person and events in the life of his community. The confession referred to history and was consciously made in history.[5]

The insight of Whitehead and Niebuhr is no less true for business ethics than for any other form of reflection on the moral significance of human action. The story of our life is the context in which we interpret our world and the basis of our action and interaction within that world. Niebuhr shows how story and history give meaning to our lives and inform collective, social moral agency as well as individual agency within community. Story is the way we express the deepest level of believing and the most powerful shaping force of our doing. Internal history pertains to our own community and tradition. External history refers to other communities and traditions, external to us but having their own internal history and story. For Niebuhr, our Christian story centers historically on Jesus Christ, through whom we have faith in the triune God who is the creator, redeemer and consummator of all histories. This God is the One whom we encounter in all the plurality of human experience, the Reality who compels us to develop and change toward our final fulfillment, the Source of the permanent revolution of all our believing and action. "This conversion and permanent revolution of our human religion through Jesus Christ is what we mean by revelation," Niebuhr concludes. "Whatever others may say we can only confess, as humans who live in history, that through our history a compulsion has been placed upon us and a new beginning offered us which we cannot evade."[6]

Narrative theology in Niebuhr's meaning, therefore, is inseparably intertwined with every aspect of human life. The ethics that humans bring to business and to the management of values in organizations is based in their history and in the story of their life no less than is the case with every other part of their lives. This is true of persons belonging to other communities of faith and to other traditions as well as to those of Christian conviction.

It is unfortunate that an ethicist like Stanley Hauerwas, who lifts up story as a means for escape from the rationalism in which he was trained, has made no use of Niebuhr's understanding of story, history and human community. In spite of his repeated mention of story, as exemplified in *Vision and Virtue*,[7] Hauerwas continues to rely, for his ethics, primarily on a rational method in which story in general and the biblical narratives in particular play only a peripheral role.

Other important resources for story-based ethics can be found in the strong, pragmatic tradition represented by Charles Sanders Peirce, William James, and Josiah Royce,[8] in the social psychology of George Herbert Mead,[9] and in the post-critical philosophy of Michael Polanyi.

The pragmatists break with the dyadic epistemology that has characterized modern Western thought and develop a triadic understanding of knowing and interpretation. For the dyadic method, the knower and the known are central; knowing is a function of an individual thinker. For the triadic method, humans emerge in community, are shaped by their communication in community, carry on the process of interpreting in community, and are constantly reshaping their understanding of themselves and their world in communal interaction. Epistemology and ontology are closely linked in the perception of traditions and communities. Interpretation is by persons in community, to others in that community of interpretation, through communication about some shared experience. Communal insight is historical, rooted in tradition and related to social location.

Mead's work establishes the social nature of selfhood. Our individuality emerges in interaction with other selves in a community of shared symbols and interpretation.

Michael Polanyi adds crucial dimensions to this perspective. A physician and physical chemist turned philosopher, Polanyi elaborates what he calls the "from-to" structure of knowing. Most attention is paid to the focus of knowing, what is affirmed as known. Polanyi shifts attention to the "tacit dimension" of knowing, to the physical, biological, social and cultural background that enables us to perceive, give attention to, interpret and affirm what we call knowledge.

For example, Polanyi's findings disclose the inadequacy of "dilemma ethics." True enough, someone may perceive an ethical dilemma confronting her or him. Yet the dilemma does not exist apart from the tacit dimension shaping the ethical perspective that enables a person to see a problem.

In a way that fits well with Niebuhr's theology and ethics, Polanyi restores the fiduciary grounding, the dimension of faith, in human knowing and acting. Polanyi writes:

> We must now recognize belief once more as the source of all knowledge. Tacit assent and intellectual passions, the sharing of an idiom and cultural heritage, affiliation to a like-minded community; such are the impulses which shape our vision of the nature of things on which we rely for our mastery of things. No intelligence, however critical or original, can operate outside such a fiduciary framework.[10]

In the centers for ethics and policy at Berkeley and elsewhere, we have shaped these resources into a covenantal or federal methodology as the basis for a story-based approach to business ethics or, as we call it, to the management of values in organizations. The word federal comes from the Latin *foedus*, which means covenant; federalism is covenantal; a covenantal view is federal. Such a methodology is very useful in Western societies as most of them are based on federal, covenantal political and social patterns. Federalism is the fastest growing political system in the twentieth century; the recent cascade of events in eastern Europe adds even more validity to this view. The federal tradition is among the most powerful theological, ethical and societal understandings pervading the modern world. In the United States especially, our political, economic and religious institutions are embued with this view. In addition, the covenant may provide a significant mode of convergence for Jewish, Protestant Christian, Roman Catholic and Eastern Orthodox ethics. Federalism has great ecumenical and interreligious potential.

Another resource for story-based ethics is the case method. Here the situation is presented in some semblance of story form. The use of cases encourages those who discuss the case to see the situation in terms of the wholeness of human experience with its complex interacting factors. It also invites those who participate in the discussion to dwell in the context of the case in community with one another.

Oliver Williams and John Houck, in *Full Value: Cases in Christian Business Ethics,* have shown how cases can relate people to the story of their own lives and thus to the Christian tradition of story. Their approach can be very helpful in the management of values.

> The Christian story would provide the images to confront the reality of the corporate world with its monetary reward system and its appeal to some of the less noble character traits of humankind. Our executive could still be exceedingly competent and successful, she could be paid well and enjoy the good things of life, but she would have an expanded vision of what her life is all about, and she would have the freedom to take a stand against some of the expectations of her corporate role. She would not be trapped in this corporate role.[11]

At the same time, we must remember that communities of policy makers in particular organizations are made up of persons from different communities of faith. A story-based approach must be broader than the perspective of one denomination and tap the depth of story present in every person and in every organizational community.

The Storied Shape of Ethics

Building on the resources mentioned above, we can begin to discern the shape of ethics as rooted in the stories of humans in community. Most important of all, in this view, ethics is not primarily what academic specialists, in philosophy or theology, do; instead, ethics is the reflection in human communities of interaction on the moral significance of human agency and deeds. That is the subject matter of ethics. Academic ethicists are doing their proper work when they explore ethics in actual human situations and illumine its meaning. In this perspective, ethics has many dimensions.

Community and Interpretation

Humans emerge from community, achieve self-conscious human identity as a part of a community, and dwell symbiotically in community. Stories are a fundamental way in which humans relate to one another, interpret themselves and their communities to one another, and shape their actions and interaction in community. The Bible is made up for the most part of narratives and recitals of varied kinds by which the

Hebrew and Christian communities understand themselves, the world as created and governed by God, and the appropriate responses they are called to make within the divine and human context. Moses and Joshua remember the story of God's deliverance of their ancestors to remind the Hebrews in each particular present whence they come, who they are, and to what covenant they are called to be faithful. The story of David, written by one of the greatest novelists of all time, shows how people and government exist under the same divine care, call and judgment. The prophets continue the covenantal narrative, calling the community to covenantal faithfulness and covenantal justice. The story of Jesus and the stories he told continue to be recounted among Christians and still shape our perspectives and actions. The same is true for other communities, for tribes in ancient Europe and present-day Africa, for nations whose history provides continuity and identity, and for organizations whose culture and character are communicated in communal stories.

Time

The story in which myth is embodied provides a sense of the past from which communities come and an understanding of the present with its relations, obligations and patterns of action. The stories of a community also give to its members an anticipated future and a sense of what is valuable in every time. The story of Arjuna before the battle does this for Hindus. The story of Buddha functions in a similar way for Buddhists, as do stories of Confucius for the community of his followers and the story of Jesus for Christians. In parallel fashion, the stories told in a corporation give oldtimers and newcomers an understanding of the company's past, present and future, with the interpretations of co-workers and expected actions this understanding provides.

Levels of Moral Agency

Stories told in human community function also to distinguish levels of responsibility and action, whereas rational methodologies tend to limit reason and agency to individuals. In the biblical narrative, God the Faithful One, who makes covenant and keeps covenant, is the primary agent in creating, judging, redeeming and bringing to consummation and fulfillment the world and its inhabitants. But nations and their rulers also act in comprehensive ways that are responsible to God's covenant and are judged by their faithfulness and unfaithfulness to that covenant, as the historical and prophetic narratives make clear. Less comprehensive communities—tribes, economic enterprises, Pharisees, Sadducees, scribes, followers of Cephas and Apollos—have characteristic, common ways of acting. Yet individuals too are agents, called to covenantal faithfulness. For purposes of organizational ethics today, we find it helpful to speak of these levels of moral action—individual, organizational, social sector, national, global and divine.

Commitment and Ownership

Stories have the capacity not only to inform but also to involve the hearers, draw them into the story, call forth commitment, and evoke ownership of the world and the responsibilities embodied in the narratives. We are aware of this capacity of well-told stories. Many historians are convinced that Richard III was one of Britain's best kings. Shakespeare's artistically great rendition of Richard as a consummate villain who murdered his nephews to get the throne, a view serving the political purposes of the Tudors who by treachery wrested the crown from Richard, continues to eclipse and triumph over careful historical research. When we go into a theater or open the covers of a novel, we enter a tacit covenant to dwell in the world the artist presents. Our commitment is such that we would not consider calling the police when we see a robbery or a murder committed on stage or in the novel. Yet we take such depth of ownership that we can weep for those whom tragedy befalls and rejoice in a happy outcome to perilous adventures. Abraham Lincoln in his Gettysburg Address tells the story of his nation, not simply to inform his hearers, but rather to summon an entire people to commitment to the great task that lies before them, "that government of the people, by the people, and for the people shall not perish from the earth." So also is it with stories in our religious communities, stories told in love and faith and so heard. Christians dwell in the story of the Good Samaritan. The commitment into which its tellers have drawn us means that we own it as our own story. We cannot, therefore, pass by anyone in need without feeling the tug to help, even though other commitments make it impossible to extend assistance in every situation. In the same way, the stories told in corporate communities call forth commitment to the organization's culture and evoke ownership of its communal values.

Change

Story also provides the basis for change in ethical perception in response to different conditions. What Niebuhr calls the permanently revolutionary nature of faith in God can be transmitted especially well through narrative. The stories are a continuously stabilizing element in communal tradition that permits the innovative aspects of creation, the new perspectives on what is redemptive and liberating, and the emerging horizons of justice and love to take their places within the evolving responses of humanity to that reality we call God in the biblical Christian community.

By contrast, ethics based upon rationality tend toward static principles and prescriptions that resist the newness of each emerging present and seem to contradict the hopefulness of humanity as we anticipate the future. In parallel fashion, human character based upon habit rather than story has a powerful tendency to maintain the injustices and oppressions of the past rather than have human character called into new visions of justice by the changes time brings.[12]

Within these dimensions, we can see that all communities and the symbiotically related individuals within them are rooted in story, narrative, history and tradition. Through commitment and ownership, communities maintain continuity of identity and interpretation throughout the interrelated levels of moral agency, yet are enabled to respond to new situations and changed conditions by means of story. On the basis of story understood in these dimensions, we move from theory to covenantal wholeness in ethics and open the way for dealing with the ethics of organizations.

A Story-Based Method for Organizational Ethics

Several interrelated purposes informed the founding of the centers for ethics and policy in Berkeley and New York and helped similar programs get started in other places in North America and Europe. The first purpose was the perceived need to supplement strategies of social change that were tied to protest with strategies internal to institutions related to policy and its implementation. Second was the purpose, related to the first, to recover the ethics of organizations from its eclipse by the focus of ethics in this century on individual ethics and ethical theory.

Third was the concern to work with policy makers in major institutions, most of whom in the United States are active participants in one religious community or another, to learn their insights about policy making and assist them in discovering the meaning of their religious convictions for their careers as policy makers, a task generally neglected by religious communities. A fourth purpose was to enrich theological education by acquainting students more closely with an important group of people with whom they would have to work in parishes when they became pastors in congregations. A fifth purpose was to contribute to the task of reshaping the organizations of modern society to serve better the concerns for human dignity, justice, quality of life and the natural order.

It became clear that resources outside ethics were essential. We adopted, therefore, what we called a triadic approach, involving persons not only from ethics but also from other academic disciplines, especially the social sciences, and from the policy arenas in centers of social dynamism. To bring these people together and to utilize the varied resources, it was necessary to develop a process of mutual learning, each group listening carefully to those from another academic or social sector to learn the different languages and dwell in the quite different perspectives. We found it necessary to work within a covenantal or federal paradigm and to develop a story-based methodology for discovering the character, the culture and values, and the tacit and explicit covenants of organizational communities.

A Federal Paradigm

Organizations are human communities, yet they are much more than a collection of individual humans. In some ways, the root metaphor[13] of a machine can be helpful in understanding organizations. The structure of organizations, viewed in rational perspective as bureaucracy, resembles a machine in its impersonal relations, rules and processes. The root metaphor of an organism also can be illuminating. The parts of an organization are distinguishable but work together interactively to form an operating whole. The root metaphor of a society also fits. People are acting and interacting through the structures of an organization. The political, economic, sociological and psychological aspects cannot be overlooked. Yet there are further dimensions that call for the root metaphor of covenant. An organization depends upon persons and groups who are involved and committed. Loyalties and convictions are at stake. There is a remembered past, a dynamic present, and an anticipated future at the core of an organization. Although a mechanical or an organic metaphor excludes the social and covenantal, and the social metaphor tends to miss the depth of faith and faithfulness that covenant includes, the covenantal or federal paradigm can include these others within itself:

> Different communities have distinct histories, diverse gods which shape their memories, their loyalties, and their hopes. While we may not be able to see how this diversity can be reduced to unity, we may draw on the resources of our different communities to accept the multiplicity of ethnic, racial, religious, and social groups. Perhaps we can even come to affirm plurality and to strengthen political and societal patterns based on less than ultimate agreement. The United States has been compelled by stubborn, irreducible social forces to fumble its way toward a form of such a pluralistic order. The federal political philosophy and the partial separation of church and state have been important elements in this development. At best, the American example is only a beginning. But it is a beginning that is being duplicated in other societies and is becoming transnational in scope. It is possible that a new humanity is moving uncertainly and haltingly toward a similar pluralism on a global scale.[14]

A federal paradigm is appropriate because the history, institutions and social patterns of the United States and most other modern Western societies are informed, shaped and imbued with federalism. It is interesting, and very unfortunate, that Alasdair MacIntyre in *After Virtue*[15] ignores, indeed seems unaware of, the pervasive and influential federal tradition. He deplores the plurality of moral visions in the modern world and longs for a lost consensus that never existed. Because he does not give attention to the federal tradition of theology, ethics and politics, the core of which is shaping plural and diverse social entities into working unities without requiring or enforcing consensus (after all, the motto of the United States is *e pluribus unum*), MacIntyre sees the only alternatives for the contemporary world to be either Nietzsche or Aristotle and obviously sees the only hope for humanity in a "return" to Aristotle. Rather than using an inaccurate, romanticized version of history and idealized hopes for the present, we need instead to build on the powerful tradition of federalism that permeates our world and which has proven quite effective in developing workable covenants among different parties, renegotiating those covenants to meet changing conditions, and serving gradually over the centuries the cause of human dignity, justice and liberation, although at a pace much slower than many of us would prefer.

Story

For a federal paradigm in which the covenants of human life form the inner meaning and empowering unity of community, a story-based method is crucial. By tapping into the rich veins of story present in corporations, it becomes possible to understand the history and character of an organization and to develop processes for renegotiating and enriching its covenants.

Since the early 1970s we have used a method permeated by story and a sense of narrative theology in its widest meaning for our organizational ethics projects conducted by the centers for ethics and policy. These projects have been with business corporations, governmental agencies, community groups of various kinds, hospitals and health care systems, churches and institutions of higher education. Though these organizations are in many ways quite distinct and the procedures in the projects differ accordingly, it is also true that every corporation is different from every other one and no health care institution is exactly like another. Given the need to adjust to the nature and needs of each organization, we have found it is possible to speak of organizational ethics, or corporate ethics in relation to businesses, and to use similar methods in our various projects. It is organizations as human communities, shaped by covenantal bonding as well as by a culture and capable of being opened through a storied method, that make it possible to handle their plurality with a relatively coherent approach.

Shaping the Project

When the possibility of a project arises, persons from the center discuss with members of senior management the need for the project, what its purposes will be and who will participate. We listen to their stories of the problems they want addressed, how they fit in with the history and purposes of the corporation, and what outcomes are wanted. In addition to developing a plan that the CEO wants and will endorse, we have a small steering committee of people who know the corporation well from inside; we arrange for an internal coordinator who generally is trusted, knows the history and character of the organization, and who is at the center of corporate communications. The center team also reads the central documents of the corporation's history and organization as a means for entering into the corporate story and culture.

Interviews

Each primary participant in the project is interviewed individually by a team consisting of an ethicist and a management scientist. The pattern of an interview represents the triadic approach and carries forward the process of mutual learning. Everyone is assured that the interviews are completely confidential, that no one will be quoted so as to identify the person, and that the material will be used to build a profile of the company which will be reported back to all participants for discussion and revision. The conversations begin, after get-acquainted time, by asking the persons how they came to be associated with the company. Without much encouragement the people tell their story. We learn a great deal about them, why they joined the organization, what it means to them, and why they have stayed. We then move on to questions about the history and character of the company, what major changes have occurred and are anticipated, how policies have evolved, what are the stakes in these shifts, the kinds of issues that seem important now, and what particular cases can be suggested for discussion in later group sessions. Without discussing ethics or values directly in any technical sense, we get answers loaded with both. In addition to the individual and corporate stories and the way these are intertwined, we build relations of trust and begin to understand and dwell in the community and covenant of this organization.

Corporate Profile

From the interviews, a profile of the culture and values of the company is derived. Value elements are identified in the interviews; the values as perceived by the interviewees are collected and ordered; clusters of values are developed; an attempt is made to discover the culture and values of the organization as reflected in the perceptions of these moral agents as they participate in the moral agency of the corporation. Particular statements and vignettes are quoted to illustrate the values and to authenticate the cultural profile derived from the interviews. It is an interesting and delicate task to organize the values in such a way as to suggest the shape of the corporate culture and to select brief statements that, as synecdoche, remind the participants of the story of their corporate life.

Small group discussions are held then, which focus on the culture and values profile as produced by the interviewers. To what extent have the participants been heard correctly? Does this statement provide a recognizable profile of this corporate community?

The statement is modified in light of these discussions to correct the misunderstandings of the interviewers. The result of this stage of the project should be a profile of the culture and values of the corporation that is organized according to the perceptions of the participants so they can recognize and affirm it. The profile has been illustrated with brief statements and vignettes suggesting situations and crucial turning points that tap into the stories of their own lives within the corporation and the story of the life of this organization.

The participants begin to realize how their individual stories relate to the corporate story, what the commitments are that underlie the organizational community, and what the tacit and explicit covenants of their life in this company are. In addition, they begin to develop a language to discuss among themselves the value dimensions of corporate policy and action, generally something they had been unaccustomed to doing. Texts and lectures by academic ethicists will, for almost all organizational executives, be in unknown tongues and, therefore, opaque. With this method they are learning ethics in their own language.

As the discussions develop, the relationship between individual moral agency and organizational moral agency becomes clearer. The levels are not merged, some tensions remain, but they are seen as closely interrelated. In addition, the discussions about the values of the company help to deepen trust among the participants as well as between them and the center personnel conducting the project.

Values Realism

Another series of discussions follows after a short interval, involving a larger number of persons than before in each group. The movement from individual interview to small groups to large groups and eventually to meetings with all participants together is deliberate and reflects their emerging ability to talk more easily with one another about the culture and values operative in their work settings.

In the next discussions, the focus is on the realism in the company's operating world and on values the participants have affirmed as forming the company's culture. Stories selected from the interviews and from discussions of the corporate profile are developed into illustrations or mini-cases dealing with values in corporate policy and action. These particular situations are explored carefully by the managers to ascertain the extent to which the actions of the company and its agents in real circumstances fit or do not fit the values previously affirmed. In the process of these discussions, the statement of culture and values can be modified further and sharpened so that it represents a more precise relating of the ethical intentions of the organization to its operational actualities. At the same time, understanding of the values is deepened and greater ownership of them is taken.

Implementation

Next, planning will be initiated to implement the realistic understanding of organizational culture and values developed. This process will involve taking the discussions beyond an upper level of managers and testing the profile at selected levels or at all levels. Usually, we train persons in the company to carry out the plan of implementation we help develop.

The approach we favor involves cascading the discussions down through the entire organization, with the culture and values statement being talked about in every workplace in a session led by the line manager in charge. An important aspect of this method revolves around getting reactions to the statement from managers and employees in every sector of the company. It is crucial to make sure that reports of the sessions as well as responses made through modification to the culture and values statement are communicated back up through the corporation's channels. By this means, it is possible for better understanding of the company's values to occur and become more operative. The opportunity to discuss this statement of company culture and values, and participate in shaping it, inevitably deepens the ownership of the values and draws people into greater support of the culture. In addition, managers and those they supervise tend to emerge from these discussions with a higher level of trust. As they discover that their own story meshes with the corporate story and that company leadership wants to receive communication as well as send it, personnel at all levels tend to identify with their work more and are willing to contribute energy and ideas toward improving the workplace and the quality of its operation. Communication up and down is improved because people feel listened to; they are willing to come up with suggestions not only about "ethical" issues but also about improvements in efficiency and productivity. This process can fit in and reinforce the development of participative styles of management.

Further steps in implementation involve working to shape the policies and actions of the corporation in every sector so they reflect more fully the company's culture and values. To accomplish this it is necessary to integrate the statement as modified into the central operations of the corporation and its every division—strategic planning, personnel, manufacturing, marketing, finance, etc. The values of the corporation as well as its technical expertise must be woven into every activity at all levels. The subjects of stories told in the company become not just founders and top executives (e.g. the "Bill and Dave" stories at Hewlett-Packard) but also ordinary managers and employees who make helpful suggestions that contribute to the entire corporate community. Stories and discussions relating to the company and the workplace become more the content of conversation and concern in off-the-job time.

As the process becomes part of the ongoing operations of the company, the intended values become clearer, are understood and owned more completely by all personnel, and are exhibited more fully in the actions of the entire corporation. Certain values will be seen as foundational in the history and life of this corporate community. Others will be identified as related to the purposes and goals of the organization. Still other values will be recognized as being especially relevant for operational processes and relations, linking the foundational and goal-related values.

In summary, trust at all levels can be increased, the communal covenants deepened, and the culture, values and covenants subtly renegotiated to become more inclusive and more realistic. As the fit of values between employees and company becomes closer, human relations and productivity are enhanced in every workplace. Most important of all, a critical dimension of ethical reflection is rendered explicit, so that the operations of the company will become better aligned with its intended values, and those values will be linked more closely to the expectations of employees and of the surrounding society.

Another way to say this is that the stories of the persons making up the company community and the story of the corporation become better integrated. Story, of course, is not the sole element in the management of values in a corporation, but it is an element at the core of the company as community and the company community as part of a larger social environment of values. A story-based method is helpful for understanding the character and culture of a corporation, for strengthening the culture, and for improving the effectiveness of management at all levels. In these ways, narrative theology and business ethics are integrally related.

Cases

At all points in the process of managing values, the case method is helpful. If cases are to be most useful, they must be cases shaped more by stories than by rational calculation, whether Kantian or utilitarian. Cases lend themselves superbly to a story-based method for managing values and teaching the management of values. Cases deal with situations of human interaction. That is the primary arena of ethics. Cases involve the wholeness of human experience rather than isolated fragments. When story is the basis, cases draw people into the human meaning of individual and organizational problems.

In the work of the centers for ethics and policy, usually we build the cases to be used in discussions on suggestions made in the interviews and subsequent sessions. They are, therefore, drawn from real occurrences within the organization. We ask for real and relevant examples but not ones that are too hot to handle at the moment.

These stories and mini-cases are also useful in writing or speaking about organizational ethics. For example, in my book *Management of Values*, each chapter opens with a condensed story. All the stories are derived from real situations, with the details changed sufficiently to protect the guilty as well as the innocent.

• • • • •

Ten senior vice-presidents of a major industrial corporation with over 200 locations scattered over the United States were meeting. The topic for discussion was how to make the corporate code and its ethics more effectively operative throughout the company.

"The real problem, as I see it," Tom was saying, "is whether we do the right thing when issues arise or do what will mean more profit. It's okay to have a code of ethics, but we are first of all in business to make money. If the profit is rolling in, we can afford to put our values into operation."

"I don't think it's that way at all," Bill replied. "We can't make a profit over the long run unless we have a strong culture with value commitments that we are always trying to practice better. One of the main reasons I like working for this company is that I believe we have values and try to build them into what we do."

Chris leaned forward in his seat. "That's what the CEO at Johnson & Johnson was saying in the videotape we saw last week. A corporation has to put the concerns of people first, or society will rebel and pass laws compelling corporations to act in approved ways."

"That was James Burke," Cliff added, joining the conversation. "He made a speech last year in New York comparing the long-term profits of corporations having strong cultures and ethical codes with corporations that did not. According to his report, it's having value commitments and practicing them throughout the company that ensures good performance."

"Well," Tom said, retreating a little, "it may be something of a chicken and egg thing. You can't tell which comes first. But I'd like some examples of how we put our ethics to work here."

"I'll give you an illustration," Frank, who had been silent up to now, said. "Last year our southwest region had just locked some of our major suppliers of raw materials into three-year contracts when the market for their products shot way up. We could have held them to the lower price legally. But I discussed it with our managers in the region, and we decided to renegotiate the contracts. We still came out well with reference to the current market but not as well as we could have in terms of the original contracts."

"If it was mushy do-gooding," Tom replied, "I'd say you were wrong. If it will turn a profit, I'd say you did right."

"I don't think those sharp alternatives are the correct ones," Frank responded. "I used to think so, but no more. The discussions we have been having over the past year about our corporate culture and ethics have given me a different perspective on the way we make decisions here. In this case we took a careful look at the different values that were involved—our long-term relations with these suppliers in the past; our plans to keep buying from them in the future; the confidence we had developed in the quality of the materials we were getting from them; the importance of their confidence in us as reliable purchasers; the times they had gone out of their way to help us and will again; and the reputation of this company in the entire region."

"It would seem to me," Bill said, "as though you looked at the trade-offs among values carefully and came up with a solution that was sound management because it combined humane values and business values."

"I agree," Bob chimed in. "I'm proud to work for a company that has those commitments. When we have similar decisions, we work them through and know that the CEO we've got will support us and so will most of the top management. Did you check with your executive vice-president before making the fnal arrangements?"

"No," Frank replied. "We included it in our reports. A note came down on that item commending us and wanting to use it as an illustration if it could be done in a way that would not embarrass anyone."

"I can think of decisions like that we've made in our division," Cliff said. "We are gradually learning that ethics is not doing something perfect but rather weighing values and working through to the best combination of trade-offs we can come up with."

"Those are illustrations of what we might call *managing values for excellence*," Bill suggested.[16]

• • • • •

The understanding of the importance of narrative theology for business ethics presented here has much to offer in work with corporations, helping them to become more aware of the value dimensions of policy and its implementation, and to bring their values and actions more into line with the environment of values in society. This story-based approach also has much to offer those who develop effective curricula of business ethics in business schools. In addition, focusing on story can be a means for creating fruitful interaction among ethicists, management scholars and business practitioners, an interaction essential for business ethics in any setting.

Notes

1.   Edith Hamilton and Huntington Cairns, eds., *The Collected Dialogues of Plato* (New York: Pantheon, 1961), pp. 607-608.

2.   Charles S. McCoy, *When Gods Change: Hope for Theology* (Nashville: Abingdon, 1980), pp. 112-113.

3.   Hans Frei, *The Eclipse of Biblical Narrative* (New Haven: Yale University Press, 1974).

4.   Mary Warnock, *Ethics Since 1900* (London: Oxford University Press, 1960, 1966, 1978), p. 144.

5.   H. Richard Niebuhr, *The Meaning of Revelation* (New York: MacMillan, 1941), pp. 43-44.

6.   *Ibid.* p. 191.

7.   Stanley Hauerwas, *Vision and Virtue: Essays in Christian Ethical Reflection* (Notre Dame, IN: Fides), 1974.

8.   See generally Hans-Otto Apel, *Der Denkweg von Charles Sanders Peirce* (Frankfurt: Suhrkamp, 1975); William James, *Pragmatism* (New York: Longmans, Green, 1907) and *A Pluralistic Universe* (New York: Longmans, Green, 1909); Josiah Royce, *The Problem of Christianity*, two volumes (New York: Macmillan, 1913); and Helmut Spinner, *Pluralismus als Erkenntnis Modell* (Frankfurt: Suhrkamp, 1974).

9.   See Anselm Strauss, ed., *The Social Psychology of George Herbert Mead* (Chicago: University of Chicago Press, 1956).

10.   Michael Polanyi, *Personal Knowledge: Towards a Post-Critical Philosophy* (Chicago: University of Chicago Press, 1958), p. 266.

11.   Oliver F. Williams and John W. Houck, *Full Value: Cases in Christian Business Ethics* (San Francisco: Harper & Row, 1978), p. 72.

12.   See generally Ernst Bloch, *Das Prinzip Hoffnung*, three volumes (Frankfurt: Suhrkamp, 1959); Juergen Moltmann, *The Theology of Hope* (New York: Harper & Row, 1967), and *The Crucified God* (New York: Harper & Row, 1974); and Polanyi, *op. cit.*, 1958.

13.   Stephen C. Pepper, *World Hypotheses: A Study in Evidence* (Berkeley: University of California Press, 1961).

14.   McCoy, *op. cit.*, 1980, pp. 52-53.

15.   Alasdair MacIntyre, *After Virtue: A Study in Moral Theory* (Notre Dame, IN: University of Notre Dame Press, 1981).

16.   Charles S. McCoy, *Management of Values: The Ethical Difference in Corporate Policy and Performance* (New York: Pitman, 1985), pp. 233-234.

Four

Religious Roots and Business Practices: Vignettes from Life

C. Samuel Calian

Scene I

"There is too much talk about ethics in business today," a candid executive declared to me as we sat in his office. "The predominate issue that daily confronts everyone," he said, "is survival." He went on to deplore the fact that "all this fuss about ethics today has diverted us from our primary task of maximizing earnings and providing jobs. Milton Friedman is right, the primary task of business is to make a profit and stay competitive."

Scene II

A business acquaintance of mine regularly attends his church's Saturday vesper service as a preparatory time of confession before Sunday's eucharistic celebration. "Why are you so faithful in your attendance?" I asked. "It's because I have more to confess than most people," he replied. "I'm in a business with fierce, ruthless competition, and I am often forced to compromise myself in order to succeed. I don't like it, but what else can I do? At the moment, I see no other choice."

Scene III

I invited a business friend to a game of racquetball. "Thanks, but no thanks," he responded. "I win in everything I set out to do. That's why I'm successful. I hate to lose, and I know I can't win at racquetball. Losing is too depressing for me; that's why I don't play."

These vignettes from life highlight the tensions in America's business society. Scene I points to the economic pressures of everyday living. Ours is a business culture where the struggle for survival receives major attention. Scene II suggests there is a religious factor that may be present for many people. Whether we are related actively or not to a religious institution is not the issue; the fact is that most individuals have some kind of faith commitment.[1] Scene III suggests that by nature we tend to be competitive; there is a strong desire "to win" in most of us. These then are three important factors of daily existence: (1) the business environment, (2) religious piety, and (3) the competitive drive to succeed. The convergence of these realities complicates life for us and makes it difficult to distinguish "right" from "wrong" when many situations seem to be a mixture of these factors. How then do we exercise responsible behavior in a free marketplace society?

Can we be profitable, religious and competitive at the same time? Is this the unspoken question confronting the religious minded in America? Have we integrated these three factors of human existence in our decision-making process? Given the competitive nature of our business society, can we be profitable without losing our souls in the process? Exactly what relationship, if any, exists between our religious roots and the economic judgments we make in our daily business affairs?

The Tension Between Survival and Ethics

To answer these questions, we need to examine further the tension between business survival and ethics described in Scene I. Is it not possible to be ethical and succeed at the same time? Businesses claim they can accomplish both objectives. Consulting recently with a successful and ethical business organization gave me the opportunity to ask the chairman of the board what, in his opinion, is the relationship of ethics to profitability? Is his company profitable because it is ethical, or is it ethical because it is profitable? What about companies that are having difficult times and feel it necessary "to cheat" on personnel, product standards, or service to survive? He answered, "Our organization is ethical because we think it is good business to be ethical." I pushed on, "But is your company above being tempted?" He hesitated and then replied, "Perhaps not, but survival at any price is not what we want in our organization. True, we haven't seriously been tested yet, but I would like to think we could maintain our principles."

This chairman of the board later admitted to me that no organization or executive can guarantee its stance, until tested. How great a price an organization or individual is willing to pay for an ethical tenet depends often upon the circumstances of the moment. A business is as ethical as its last transaction. Through the media sometimes we learn the details of a questionable past transaction which may compromise the ethical image of our favorite company.

Business and ethics are not only dependent upon each other; in large measure they help to define each other. Charles W. Parry, chairman and chief executive officer of Alcoa, expresses the relationship as follows:

> Business is not separate from society. It is not an ethical adversary of the common good. Instead, business is a reflection of society. It is the method by which individuals unite to form a network of common interest. Ethics is not something businessmen must violate in order to make a profit; it is something they must implement in order to prevent chaos.[2]

The ethics of a business organization is subject constantly to attack and unexpected developments. Businesses always can declare their firm determination to be ethical but, until they are tested, we never know exactly how faithfully these ethical standards are maintained. In an imperfect world, there appears to be no such thing as a perfect ethical decision. Trade-offs are inescapable. Each new situation presents another challenge; such are the dynamics of the marketplace. Codes of ethics in operation today will not minimize the challenges we confront. The successful past history of an ethical company is always under pressure to uphold its positive image before the public.

How an organization handles the tension between survival and ethics is a significant clue to the ethical life-style of that organization. To boast too loudly about the ethics of one's organization can become embarrassing in light of subsequent disclosures. My own feeling is that companies ought to soften their ethical claims, realizing that the practice of business, far from being ideal, is more or less as ethical as the insecurities of the marketplace dictate at any given time. Such an admission is more than many businesses are willing to confess, even to themselves. No one likes to see oneself as being unethical in the marketplace. We prefer to consider ourselves ethical; public relations firms are paid handsomely to communicate a positive public image. Once the public image of a company has been besmirched, there is no quick recovery for that firm. It should not surprise us then that businesses are defensive each time some critical comment or event surfaces. Because we are not living in a perfect world, nor are we pure, an organization is prudent to avoid the self-righteous trap. A more realistic appraisal of our world and human nature is needed if we are to begin to become ethically effective and responsible in the marketplace.

The relentless pressures to survive in our society are demanding. Keyed to self-interest and paranoid feelings, they condition us to (1) look out for number one; (2) break promises when expedient; (3) trust no one; (4) hide personal errors; (5) win and retain power by any means; (6) subvert the law; (7) suppress generosity; (8) affix a price on everyone and everything; and (9) stress loyalty over truth. If survival demands that we adopt these attitudes, what room is there for a more humane ethic? If this is reality, then the best preparation is to develop tough-mindedness and leave ethics to churches, synagogues and academies. If this is not the best of all worlds, it is at least the only world we have. Let us not delude ourselves into a frame of idealism that does not exist. Life is difficult; our basic vocation is to be realistic. How can we be realistic and humanly responsible to one another?

Is There an Ethic for Competition?

Before we can build any virtuous model, we must acknowledge with regret that present conditions encourage cheating in countless ways to win at any cost. Many persons see no viable alternative and seek escape some day from this dreaded "rat race" through utopic retirement. On the other hand, if we are among the winners, our existence may not seem so bad; we continue the struggle and manage to be on the winning side most of the time. As a consequence, we refrain from criticizing or blowing the whistle in the face of unfair acts and wrong-doing so long as we are not affected personally. We prefer to remain ignorant of questionable decisions and actions in the organization. Unfortunately, and too often, this kind of naivité is erased finally by personal shocks of displacement, firing, etc.

In the meantime, each of us harbors within ourselves an individual filter system that creates reality for us. Each filter system is a mysterious blend of fiction and nonfiction: observations, experiences and myths.

We change only the mix when we are forced to confront an unexpected and unpleasant crisis; in this evaluation, we discover our naivité. A realistic ethic must challenge and expose the human situation more accurately than we have done through our individual filter systems. It must have a sufficient overview of our existence and describe it to us without delusion.

Ethics and survival need not be in opposition. The prerequisite for a workable free enterprise system is the upholding and enforcement of an ethical environment which is applied uniformly and fairly to all parties. Without a monitored ethical environment, we can expect the competition to become more intensified and our existence less human. Good intentions and carefully worded codes of ethics are not enough if an organization suspects that a competitor is taking unfair advantage through unethical practices. How long can a person or company remain ethical when other modes of operation surround them? This question is often heard in the marketplace.

If ethics are to prevail in the marketplace, the responsibility for development must not be limited to the efforts of executive management. The process must engage all persons concerned. There needs to be a genuine sense of ownership among management, employees, shareholders and even competitors. Such total involvement serves the mutual welfare of all and avoids the "dog-eat-dog" existence so often encountered in the marketplace. An ethical consciousness based upon a widening circle of ownership and enlightened self-interest has the potential for being enforced and regulated. In this way the quality of life in the business community will improve as a more humane ethic develops for a competitive world.

How does this process get started? And by whom? Such important questions need to be tackled by a coalition of committed citizens who represent all major aspects of our society. Our Center for Business, Religion, and the Professions at Pittsburgh Theological Seminary serves as an important catalyst for forming coalitions of responsible leaders in communities acting together to enhance the quality of life for all.

The Quality of Life and Religious Underpinnings

An essential question for our Center for Business, Religion, and the Professions is whether there is any consensus on virtues pointing to a satisfying "quality of life." Can some quantitative and qualitative measurements for our well-being be reached? Beyond material measurements for the quality of life, there exist intangible values (virtues) which keep us human— love, friendship, fulfillment, freedom and flexibility, good family relations, and the excitement in pursuing an idea or project. Underlying this list is a person's own feeling of respect for himself or herself and others. More often than not, our religious commitments contribute and nurture this respect for self and others. The businessman mentioned in Scene II of our beginning discussion found solace in religion to heal his damaged self-respect and guilt in the midst of numerous business pressures.

As I reflect further on Scene II, I realize that this businessman was faced with something more than a question of business ethics. He was struggling to have an honest relationship between his business and his religion. How did he envision this relationship? Did his religion serve to soothe his guilt feelings? Was his confession an admission that he knows the difference between right and wrong, but cannot help himself? Did he want God not only to forgive him but to empathize with his situation? Or are business decisions amoral? One business executive reasoned with me, "Business judgments are measured in terms of their usefulness to produce goals to ensure economic survival. Thus business dealings are not subject to moral evaluations; miscalculations and wrong decisions do not constitute guilt for which it would be necessary to seek forgiveness." Is that true?

The businessman in Scene II sees himself as a religious person who ought to be neither praised nor damned, but understood. His faith has given him insight into himself and human nature in general. He wants to maintain a quality of life that is both material and spiritual in content. He considers himself a sinner in need of constant renewal. The interplay between his business and religion is highlighted in the confessional process practiced in his life. He finds himself in an unending tension, belonging to two worlds at the same time. He has learned to accept the unresolved demands of the interplay as his personal "cross." Apparently, he prefers this route rather than rationalizing his shortcomings or soothing his guilt through various forms of psychological relief. He feels he is doing wrong and, without any excuses for himself, openly seeks Divine forgiveness. Yet, at the same time, he believes he cannot conduct his business otherwise if he wishes to survive.

Faced with this dilemma, what advice can we offer that is neither moralistic nor unrealistic? How can he succeed at his business and remain faithful to the standards of his faith at the same time? The quality of life for him is both material and spiritual, and herein lies his deeper problem.

Basic Roles of Business and Religion

Has this businessman confused the basic roles of business and religion? Businesses are essentially profit oriented, the means of livelihood for the entrepreneur, employer and employee. A successful business provides the monies necessary to live, to enjoy good health, and to satisfy basic concerns for a fulfilled life. Ours is a business culture. However, we need to remind ourselves that business is not the *raison d'être* of our lives: it ought to be the means of life. Is there not more to life than running through the numbers? Business provides the wherewithal to obtain material goods, and serves as an instrument for us to reach our goals and agendas in life. Religion, unlike business, stands for what is ultimate in life. The religious vision ought to question the *status quo* operations of daily life. It points us to the end for which we are striving—our aspirations, expectations and dreams. The religious vision judges the content of our living, and reveals our nakedness. It singles out what goals are short-sighted and unworthy of our devotion.

There is always the danger that our business will become our religion. When the means becomes the end, we are in danger of losing our self-respect, defacing the image of God in us and in others. Authentic religion warns against this danger: it informs us of the consequences of worshipping a golden calf. To see this process taking over our lives and to do nothing is hell. Life is more than a series of deals, otherwise everyone and everything would become a means to an end. To avoid this, my business acquaintance was attempting to maintain an uncomfortable interplay between his religion and his business. Whether he will be able to sustain the interplay is another question. To avoid the effort would open even wider the doors of idolatry, producing only more golden calves empty of love and forgiveness.

There have been those also who have turned their religion into a business, making the former a profitable commodity filled with false promises that later leave individuals dismayed and disappointed. Here again, the healthy tension between means and end has been distorted and even destroyed. To prevent this, we need to separate the task of business and the purpose of religion. At all costs, we must avoid the temptation of baptizing either into the image of the other. We need to lift up the essential integrity of each if the relationship is to be vital and beneficial. Instinctively, this is what my business acquaintance sought as he confessed his shortcomings during the weekly vesper services. He was seeking to overcome the temptation of cheap rationalizations for his behavior or psychological accommodations that might dull the hard realities of life.

A good relationship between business and religion is one in which the separate visions and concepts of reality are recognized. None of us can afford to live a one-dimensional existence. The means of livelihood and the transcendent dimensions of life must be related. Preoccupied only with business, we can come to regard the profit and loss column as the ultimate reality of our existence. How sterile our lives then become! At the same time, an obsession with a spiritualized religion likewise can pervert our perspective and deafen us to the present struggles of individuals. Religious reality informs us that our identities and destinies are far more important than any immediate trade-off that might rob us of integrity and vision for a better tomorrow. A living faith will keep the cutting edge of that concern before us without compromise.

The biblical witness, nurtured through my Christian understanding, reminds me that the primary end of life is always to give honor to God in whose image we are created. Honoring God implies honoring my neighbor as well, since the latter also is created in God's image. There is no justifiable reason to dishonor either God or neighbor. Since this standard is too high for most of us, we find ourselves in need of confessing our shortcomings regularly. The truth is that no one can go through a week of living before God and neighbor without forgiving and being forgiven. Unfortunately however, ours is a vengeful and suspicious society. The human community is largely unforgiving: We remember and scorn the shortcomings of others as they have affected us. To forgive and be forgiven should be a constant transaction if we are to stay in touch with each other's humanity. The interplay between our faith and our practices reminds us of this reality. *But is there room for forgiveness in a business world?* This question confronts us in our desire to be realistic. To forgive implies risk taking and cost: The price may be too high for some.

When business is viewed as a means, we realize that no short-term gains are worth the price of losing our self-respect or respect for others.

Religion challenges us to be less near-sighted, to take a broader view in our day-to-day struggles. Religious commitment, within the Judeo-Christian spectrum, is not escapist oriented; it is willing to face the daily skirmishes and battles of the marketplace. Our faith enables us to expand our vision toward a transcendent perspective which entails suffering. The fact of suffering is an inescapable issue facing the businessman in Scene II. So far, he has refused to follow his faith completely; the weekly vesper service consequently reminds him that he has been a loser before God. Is he willing to pay the price involved to carry, if you will, his cross all the way? Religious commitments do not come cheaply; they shape virtuous behavior with essential principles to keep human life human.

There will always exist a tension, then, between religious beliefs and business practices; through the struggle we can sort out the issues involved, without destroying the essential nature of either. Business and religion must not be lumped in the same image, but must be viewed in their separate natures if creative dialogue and cooperation are to take place. Means and end are inextricably related, and in the final analysis both need to be reviewed in the light of a Higher Agenda witnessed in the Scriptures.

The Issue of Winning

Early in our discussion we raised the question, Can we be profitable, religious and competitive at the same time? We need now to say a further word about competition, since it raises for us the issue of winning or "making it" in society. Remember my business friend in Scene III, who refused to play racquetball? Is he typical of today's business community? The hope for success and the fear of failure are perhaps the two greatest burdens people carry on their shoulders today. We seem to be looking for some secret formula to usher us into the winner's circle on a permanent basis. No one is beyond the magnetism of winning, even when we pretend otherwise.

On the other hand, nothing fails like success. The more successes one achieves, the greater the addiction becomes. A winning streak can become a diabolical chain that nurtures and contributes to our anxieties, restlessness and sense of incompleteness. In short, too much success may be dangerous to our health and sense of wholeness.

The person who lacks the courage to admit imperfections and experiences of losing is forced to deal in appearances. To maintain a pretense of winning is a facade, a false front. This mask contributes to the identity crises of individuals who appear as winners while actually losing in their search for authentic selfhood.

The confession of sins in the liturgy of the Christian church is not a *pro forma* exercise. It is a confession of human failings, helping us to maintain our perspective. God does not expect perfection, nor does God demand winners. When imperfection (sin) is taken seriously, the burden of perfectionism is removed. God knows we are not perfect; everyone's life is tainted with failure. Self-respect and self-esteem from a Judeo-Christian perspective are not based on successes in society; our worth is measured by the quality of our relationships with God and each other. From the biblical perspective, any victory at the price of a broken relationship is really a loss. To understand this concept is to be liberated from the win/lose structures of our culture which often victimize us and our families. This is a difficult lesson to communicate to a competitive marketplace greedy to win.

Life is more than an enlarged scoreboard to record wins and losses. Life does not require us to win; it asks us instead to grow. Our losses can nurture us as well as our successes. From the vantage point of my Christian heritage, we humans are life-long pilgrims, stewards before God who has given us the gift of life we enjoy. This gift *grows* in meaning with every experience, and growth is primarily nurtured through relationships. Hence the importance placed on human ties with one another; to endanger these ties is to be a loser in life no matter how much you win in material terms. Unlike our competitive culture, which rushes to anoint its winners during their lifetime, the church declares its saints posthumously. The church is aware that its saints are simply sinners revised and edited.

The Decision-Making Process

Religion today essentially informs and prepares the basic framework for virtuous behavior for a large percentage of people in the business community. Yet, in practice how close is the relationship between one's religious roots and business practices? Exactly how does the decision process unfold in business?

From surveys and study, I find that decision makers wish to approach the marketplace realistically. Survival and self-interest, therefore, are paramount concerns in a marketplace that recognizes the necessity for compromise and trade-offs. Thus, it is important for decision makers always to decide what is negotiable and what is nonnegotiable from the vantage point of our values in life. Trade-offs are inevitable; however, in retrospect we might discover that, at times, we have paid too high a price financially and morally. In our private moments we confess to ourselves that *we are at best imperfect individuals, trying to make imperfect decisions in an imperfect world.* Attempting to structure an ethical framework fortified and nurtured by our religious roots, I believe, becomes essential when our human situation is viewed realistically.

In practice, it seems our business judgments seldom are consciously formed by our religious convictions (see Executive Ethics Questionnaire in Appendix). Instead, we are largely conditioned by a reasoning process that usually asks the following set of questions: (1) Will this decision serve the best interests of the business? (2) Is it legal? (3) Does it promote a fair return? (4) Will the product or service fulfill a need? Inevitably, the answers will determine the trade-off to be made as a careful balancing act is maintained and later explained as company policy. The extent to which ethics are injected into the conversation is limited normally to the questions of legality—an area that often provides flexible interpretations.

However, ethics are more than legality; they are a commitment to a style of doing business based upon the intrinsic worth of individuals and an explicit hierarchy of values that gives substance to the company's self-image. The marketplace pressures to survive and win are sufficiently great to undermine any company's good intentions, hence the need to build upon a realistic assessment and enforcement policy that will prevail in times of pressure. Being ethical is not cheap. There is a cost involved. As there are "no free lunches," there are also no "free rides" in the pursuit of being virtuous. There is always a price tag in every ethical exchange. Ethics as a costly affair may create tensions with the profitability projections of a company—a test that many a struggling business can ill afford. Many businesses, of course, have been at both ends of the economic spectrum, experiencing good times as well as bad, and know how dehumanizing winning (struggling to get to the top) or losing (hoping to keep one's job) can be. Ours is a competitive system of doing business, and this ups and downs effect is part of the price we have agreed to pay for free enterprise. In moments of weakness, we are tempted to cheat on the system. The end result is detrimental to our freedom and way of doing business. This has been the underlying message of Ralph Nader for years.

Competition also reveals human nature to us. Adam Smith pointed this out long ago when he advised that we should allow ample room for our respective self-interests to have free play and so be productive and mutually beneficial to one another. Smith knew that we are all hungry to succeed and serve individual self-interest, and that some are more successful than others in grabbing a bigger share of the market. Marketplace realities are based upon the propensity to be greedy, not generous, in our dealings.

The executive ethics survey (see Appendix) I conducted, asked business leaders, How do you understand the phrase "business is business"? The respondents could answer: "anything goes," "money talks," "everyone has a price," "don't expect generosity," "other." The majority interpreted the phrase to mean "do not expect generosity." This may explain why, later in life, some business executives seek to soften their earlier image through philanthropy.

This tendency toward greediness and monopoly is more than self-serving; it reveals our characteristic practice to trade off precious relationships if we must, to cheat if this will ensure a win, and to lie when necessary for the sake of one's interest or enterprise. Unfortunately, like the Great Gatsby, we seem bent on rationalizing and even assuming fictional practices; we are shocked, therefore, when we read in the newspapers or view on television the extent of our inhumanity toward one another, not only in times of war but in the daily battlefields of the marketplace. I believe our inability or refusal to face the reality of our human nature is a major reason why codes of ethics and all forms of legality will not prove adequate to establish trust and confidence in the business community.

The vast majority of the respondents to my executive questionnaire interestingly enough saw themselves as being religious. When asked, Do your religious beliefs have impact on the way you actually do business? they replied overwhelmingly that religion does have an important impact on their business practices. This was expressed also to me numerous times during the thirteen weeks I participated in the Advanced Management Program at the Harvard University Graduate School of Business with 130 business executives. Yet, how close a correlation actually exists between religious roots and daily business operations may never be known, I suspect, with certainty.

"Ten Commandments" for the Marketplace

To assist businesses in their desire to be ethical, certain biblical guidelines can be given to sharpen business judgments confronted by ambiguous situations. They are as follows:

1. *Treat individuals as sacred*; people are more than means to another's end.
2. *Be generous*; the benefits will exceed the cost in the long term.
3. *Practice moderation*; obsession with winning is dehumanizing and idolatrous.
4. *Disclose mistakes*; confession and restitution are necessary means to restoring ethical character.
5. *Arrange priorities*; have long-range goals and principles in mind.
6. *Keep promises*; trust, confidence, and authenticity are built over a period of time.
7. *Tell the truth*; falsifying information destroys credibility.
8. *Exercise a more inclusive sense of stewardship*; charity does not stop at home but extends throughout our global-oriented society.
9. *Insist on being well informed*; judgment without knowledge is dangerous.
10. *Be profitable without losing your soul in the process*; evaluate your Profit and Loss Statement in light of your trade-offs—a business audit is much more than an accounting of dollars and cents.

Translating these biblical insights and principles into codes of ethics and company policies can move us toward humanizing the marketplace. In practice, we may be able only to practice approximations of these standards but, as guidelines, they serve as vital benchmarks in today's marketplace. In addition, those who practice ethically motivated leadership and who feel isolated can establish support groups to improve daily operations, encourage efficiency, heighten listening and respect for others—all characteristics of successful companies that desire a healthy future.

Conclusion

A virtuous life and leadership do indeed bring benefits to an organization, but they are also costly. To indicate otherwise is to deceive ourselves. At the same time, the need to survive is fundamental; its demand can never be ignored without detriment to the business. There will always exist, therefore, an inevitable tension between economic survival and virtuous practice.

If immediate survival is pitted against virtue, the latter will often lose given our basic instinct for self-preservation. On the other hand, any executive, employee or shareholder fearful of paying too high a price for a virtuous life needs to be challenged. Our tendency is to be myopic regarding our individual and collective self-interest. What meaning is there in surviving on this economic ship of ours if we are scrambling and killing each other in a futile attempt to reach shore? The choice is ours to make: to succeed at whatever the price or to accept the cost of being virtuous based on religious roots. Trade-offs may be inevitable in our efforts to be profitable, religious and competitive at the same time. Frankly, we must extend and broaden our understanding of succeeding beyond our immediate desire to win, as we distinguish skirmishes from battles in our business practices. Finally, let us aim to give ourselves selectively to those struggles that clearly honor God and promote virtuous living.

Notes

1. My own faith commitment has been influenced by the emphases found in John Calvin who pioneered the Reformed Tradition and reforming spirit expressed in the *Book of Confessions* of the Presbyterian Church (U.S.A.).

2. Charles W. Parry, "My Company—Right or Wrong?" *The Corporate Board*, from *The Journal of Corporate Governance*, January/February 1986, p. 20.

Appendix

Executive Ethics Questionnaire

The questionnaire is designed to understand the decision process and ethical content of business judgments. To what extent is business leadership ethically motivated, and what nurtures and sustains these ethical views? Is there a correlation between religious roots and ethical practices in business? The complete data gathered from this questionnaire are still subject to further study and investigation.

The questionnaire was sent regionally to smaller businesses in the northern Midwest and then mailed nationally to the larger 1000 companies normally listed in *Fortune*. The response to the two-page questionnaire was good, compared to a predicted average of 10 percent response for such surveys. Out of the 2,548 questionnaires sent, 492 replied, for an overall 19 percent response. The national mailing was sent to chief executive officers and vice presidents of sales and marketing. Respondents were asked to answer anonymously (and most did), and the questionnaire was coded for separation of various categories which will serve as the basis for additional interpretive analysis.

As a recent participant in the Advanced Management Program at the Harvard University Graduate School of Business, I asked the business executives present if they would also like to participate in the survey. Thirty percent of the class responded affirmatively; their replies, for the most part, were similar to the responses of the national survey. (Where there is a difference, I have made a notation on the questionnaire.)

Instead of indicating a numerical breakdown to each question, I will simply mark the preference of the majority of respondents; a strong minority reaction also has been noted. Finally, I am of the opinion that such surveys are less than scientific, but they are useful tools for conversation and consideration among members of the business and professional communities.

1) In your experience has the chief executive set the ethical climate?
    ____ completely; _X_ considerably; ____ minimally; ____ none.

2) How is the ethical climate in your organization upheld? _X_ regulations;
    _X_ trusting atmosphere; ____ rewards and punishments; ____ other.
    (Almost an equal number in each category.)

3) How do you regard your organization or business to be ethical?
    Because: ____ product is beneficial for people; ____ means of
    production considers well-being of employees; ____ production process
    does not endanger health; ____ wages are good; _X_ all of these;
    other _____ .

4) Are most codes of ethics superficial or meaningful to a business organization? ___ mostly superficial; _X_ mostly meaningful; ___ if other, explain.

5) Do you think that colleges and universities should offer a course devoted entirely to business ethics? _X_ yes; ___ no; _X_ ethics incorporated into existing courses. (AMP Class)

6) What do you think of Lombardi's famous saying: "Winning isn't everything; it's the only thing"? ___ agree; _X_ agree to a large extent; ___ agree slightly; ___ disagree.

7) Has your company engaged in a recent event of ethical consequence of which you feel especially proud? Describe. (There were many illustrations given.)

8) When does salesmanship become bribery? ___ inexpensive "give-aways" (rulers, letter openers, etc); ___ moderate "give-aways" ___ (tickets to plays or ball games, lunches, Christmas bottle of Scotch); _X_ expensive gifts (vacation trips, etc.); ___ other.

9) How would you describe the <u>process</u> by which you make ethical decisions? Rank the following from 1 (most important) through to 6 (least important).
<u>1</u> common sense   <u>4</u> self-interest
<u>2</u> what the law specifies <u>5</u> company interest   <u>6</u> Golden rule
<u>3</u> religious principles (i.e., love, justice, forgiveness, etc.)
__ other (specify)   (AMP would have self-interest as a "3.")

10) Would you suffer a career setback or other subtle management retaliation if in a specific situation you put personal standards ahead of the company's expectations, and the management felt that business suffered somehow because of it? ___ probably; _X_ probably not. (AMP were divided equally in each category.)

11) If business is a game to be won or lost, should the ethics of business be seen in terms of right and wrong strategies and not in terms of absolute standards of justice, honesty, loyalty, etc.? ___ yes; _X_ no; ___ uncertain.

12) Does an ethical posture improve or impede your company's business efficiency? _X_ improve; ___ impede; ___ if other, explain.

13) Does customer cheating make it difficult for you to maintain your own ethical posture? ___ completely; ___ substantially; _X_ moderately; _X_ very little; ___ not at all. (Almost an equal number in each category.)

14) Is it possible to agree on a common standard of values in our society? ____ completely possible; __X__ highly probable; __X__ perhaps; __X__ unlikely; ____ impossible. (Respondents were split three ways.)

15) Can you be honest, profitable, and socially responsible <u>at the same time</u> in your business dealings? __X__ yes; ____ no. Explain.

16) What is your view of human nature? Persons are: __X__ basically good; __X__ good most of the time; ____ bad most of the time; ____ basically bad. (Respondents picked both categories.)

17) Do you feel the present ethical consciousness of your business community is adequate? __X__ yes; ____ no. If <u>no</u>, explain. (There was a significant minority of "no" respondents.)

18) Do your religious beliefs have impact on the way you actually do business? ____ entirely; __X__ to a high degree; ____ slightly; ____ not at all; ____ I do not regard myself as religious.

19) Does your company support what it says about the importance of product quality and customer service? __X__ yes (describe process); ____ in a limited way; ____ no. (There were many descriptions of the process involved.)

20) How do you understand the phrase "business is business"? ____ anything goes; ____ money talks; ____ everyone has a price; __X__ don't expect generosity; ____ other.

21) Who on the current national scene is your personal model of an ethical business person? (Give person's name and business.) <u>Many names were submitted; no consensus.</u>

22) Do you believe that an ethical code established by your company makes it stronger and more profitable? __X__ in all cases; __X__ in some cases; ____ no. Explain. (AMP Class)

23) You are caught in a conflict between accepted business standards at home and prevailing practices overseas. What do you do? __X__ adapt to the demands of the situation; __X__ risk the loss of business; ____ follow the patterns already set by your competitors; ____ other. (AMP class was divided between adapting to the situation and risking the loss of business.)

24) What is your motivation to be ethical? Rank the following from 1 (most important) to 4 (least important). __1__ reason; __2__ compassion; __4__ fear of God; __3__ threat of being sued; ____ other.

25)   Should religious institutions do more to help clarify practical ethical issues? _X_ yes; ___ no. Explain. (A significant minority replied "no" in opposition to boycotts and shareholder resolutions organized by religious groups.)

26)   What is your religious affiliation? _X_ Protestant; _X_ Catholic; _X_ Orthodox; _X_ Jewish; _X_ Muslim; _X_ other. What basic beliefs guide your daily decisions. (Virtually everyone claimed some religious affiliation.)

Five

The Corporate Executive's Dharma: Insights from the Indian Epic Mahabharata

Krishna S. Dhir

Corporations clearly have obligations to their stockholders and, by and large, these are fiduciary responsibilities that arise from ownership by persons or institutions. However, the separation of ownership from control has produced a set of enigmatic problems, labeled collectively as "The Corporation Problem." The "corporation problem" relates to the corporate executive's decision-making behavior, and includes issues of (a) *efficiency* in corporate management (i.e., whether the decision-making behavior yields the greatest return to the organization or to the owners), (b) the vitiating effects of corporate *bureaucracy*, and (c) the legitimacy of corporate hierarchy. In this chapter, insights offered by the great Indian epic, the *Mahabharata*, in regard to such decision-making behavior are discussed. The evolution of the factors that resulted in the separation of corporate ownership and corporate control is first briefly traced and then the theory of *dharma* or virtuous and righteous conduct offered by the Hindu religious and philosophical literature is introduced. In the *Mahabharata*, the "corporation problem" is described in the context of "a husband's supremacy over his wife," or the lack thereof, rather than the corporate executive's supremacy over stockholders, employees, creditors, etc. This description provides a flavor of how the Indian philosophic thought would treat the corporate executive's "corporation problem."

Separation of Ownership and Control

The late nineteenth century saw many dramatic developments in the conduct of economic activity in the United States. Perhaps the most spectacular was the emergence of large-scale manufacturing. After the severe depression of 1873, the nature of business transformed from light to heavy industry. Mass production generated economies of scale and, to realize such economies, business organizations had to be large. Mass production also required mass consumption. Firms that previously were engaged only in manufacturing also took on the marketing and other functions. With growth in size and complexity of the vertically integrated firm, the need for expert advice and administrative structure became evident.

The firm became too large for one person, the owner, to manage and soon a group of executives managed each large firm. The organization was highly centralized, with a number of departments. Firms also underwent legal transformation; the use of corporate charter increasingly replaced partnerships. The corporation offered limited liability to individual owners who could sell or transfer their shares to others without disturbing the business operation. More importantly, the corporate structure allowed access to a larger pool of capital funds through the sale of stocks and bonds.

Firms began to buy stocks in other firms. Mergers and acquisitions followed. Single-product, single-function firms evolved into multi-product, multi-function businesses. The diversification movement led electric machinery manufacturing companies into appliance markets, meat packers into the manufacture of soap, and automobile manufacturers into producing refrigerators. The managers soon realized that diversified organizations required a different managerial approach. During the 1920s, DuPont, General Motors, Sears Roebuck and Standard Oil were among the first to decentralize their organizations.[1]

Ownership was separated from control as soon as ownership became distributed through shares that could be bought and sold on the stock market. Even if the shareholders were inclined and able to tackle the many intricate decisions involved in running the multi-product, multi-function, mass production-based business operation, they could not do so. The practical considerations of the logistics involved were forbidding.

Similarly, one person could not manage the complexities and decision-making challenges of a large-scale enterprise. Specialists were sought who could deal with capital budgeting, marketing, labor and personnel relations, production, engineering, etc. This division of labor resulted in the decision-making authority being vested more and more in a group of career executives who had little ownership stake in the company they managed. The owners were no longer in control. The professional executive's role was to act as an arbitrator for the collective enterprise in which the management, owners, creditors, vendors, employees, competitors, consumers and government had interests; this called for the broadening of motives and objectives of the business enterprise.

The Issue of Legitimacy

There are those who are critical of the power of the modern corporate executive who exercises control over other people's resources. The critics insist that the executive has no legitimacy, having been neither elected nor appointed and, therefore, is not responsible to anyone. The implication is that, in the nineteenth century, the question of legitimacy did not arise because the executive was also the owner. A major source of dissatisfaction is the compensation paid out to corporate executives. The managers of the most successful corporations are not necessarily the highest paid, and generous stock options and salaries have not necessarily produced stellar corporate performances in terms of sales and earnings.

According to some critics, the modern corporate management is motivated by a desire to perpetuate itself as a bureaucratic oligarchy. To back their claim, the critics point to corporate response to takeover attempts: The strategies adopted to prevent hostile takeovers are not necessarily in the stockholders' interests. Administration of poison pills, deliberate acquisition of liability, and other actions intended to make the takeover target unattractive to a raider, generally protect the management's job at the expense of lowering the stockholders' value. Such strategic moves by a corporate executive prevents the stockholders from maximizing their gains.

On the other hand, the raiders also come under fire. Takeovers are supposed to function in the interest of the stockholders. They are supposed to shake up overly complacent managers and bring about useful organizational restructuring and efficient resource deployment. Instead, hundreds of deals are made for the sake of profits on paper and for the fees and stock payoffs they generate, distracting corporate America from its real work of improving products and services. Today, corporate America is heavily debt ridden. In 1986 alone, 3,973 takeovers, mergers and buy-outs were completed at a record total cost of $236 billion.[2]

Alfred P. Sloan, Jr., wrote in October 1927:

> There is a point beyond which diffusion of stock ownership must enfeeble the corporation by depriving it of virile interest in management upon the part of some one man or group of men to whom its success is a matter of personal and vital interest. And conversely at that same point the public interest becomes involved when the public can no longer locate some tangible personality within the ownership which it may hold responsible for the corporation's conduct.[3]

Although the modern executive may be freer from the owner's control, he or she does, in fact, have constraints such as competition, customers, rival products, labor unions, public opinions, regulators in the government, and other executives within the corporate world. As the Telephone Company's Theodore N. Vail, a proponent of government regulation and an opponent of government ownership, said in 1912:

> There are few big captains of industry who can run a great corporation, but there are any quantity of men who could review their acts and who...could say whether or not the men who were doing things were doing them right.[4]

Nevertheless, public opinion is against corporate America today. In a TIME/CNN poll taken in February 1990, 68 percent of those polled regarded mergers and takeovers as "not a good thing" for the U.S. economy, and 74 percent regarded the corporate debt piled up in the 1980s to be a "serious" or "very serious" problem for the 1990s.[5]

Moral Dilemma and the Corporate Executive

As indicated in the flyer from the University of Notre Dame Center for Ethics and Religious Values in Business, announcing the symposium on "A Virtuous Life in the Business Story," contemporary discussion on the ethics and moral obligation of corporate decision making has been "dominated by the two major theories of principle, the deontological and the utilitarian." The deontological approach studies the corporate decision-making behavior in terms of binding obligations, as in duty. The utilitarian approach studies this behavior in the tradition of Bentham, stressing the importance of utility over beauty or other considerations. As pointed out in the flier, decision-making behavior demonstrated "in the *courage* to act in protecting human welfare even in the midst of incomplete information, and in the *integrity* and *humility* in communicating with consumers about possible difficulties with a product" is not explained by these approaches. These theories fall short of explaining behavior emanating from considerations of virtue.

An alternative theory, one which may well be regarded as the Universal Theory of Virtue, is offered in the Hindu religious and philosophical literature. Central to this theory is the concept of *dharma* or virtuous and righteous conduct. This concept enables us to re-examine the nature of corporate morality and moral dilemma. The problem is particularly interesting because morality is not an Indian concept. Its Sanskrit equivalent is not easy to discover. One finds "only a strict status compartmentalization of private and social ethics."[6] In the Hindu philosophic literature, nearest to the concept of morality is the ubiquitous and enigmatic concept of *dharma.*

Stories in classical and contemporary Hindu religious literature, however, are rich in accounts of moral dilemmas, most of which remain unresolved. Basically, these dilemmas arise when the agent faces two or more obligations, but circumstances are such that fulfillment of one violates one, some or all the other obligations. The decision maker is faced with irreconcilable alternatives. The actual choice among the alternatives becomes either irrational or based on grounds other than morals. Moral philosophers usually have denied that such dilemmas are possible. An adequate moral theory is supposed to eliminate them; that is to say, such dilemmas are not genuine. Kant, for instance, states:

> Because...duty and obligations are, in general, concepts that express the objective practical necessity of certain actions, and because two mutually opposing rules cannot be necessary at the same time, then it is a duty to act according to one of them, it is not only a duty but contrary to duty to act according to the other.[7]

Indian thought takes issue with Kant's claim, as illustrated in the *Bhagavad-Gita.* This is an account of Arjuna's moral dilemma, and Krishna's analysis of Arjuna's dilemma. The keeping of a promise, for instance, is a strong obligation, regarded as equivalent to being truthful or even protecting the truth. Plato has described an instance of dilemma "in which the return of a cache of weapons has been promised to a man who, intent on mayhem, comes to claim them."[8] Here, a conflict is created between two opposing principles: that of keeping a promise and that of benevolence; that of truth and that of non-violence. In Kantian ethics, truth telling gets the highest priority. In the *Bhagavad-Gita*, however, Krishna argued that promise keeping or even truthfulness cannot be an unconditional obligation when it is in conflict with the avoidance of grossly unjust and criminal acts such as patricide and fratricide. Saving an innocent life is also a strong obligation. Thus, two almost equally strong obligations or duties (*dharmas*) are in conflict here, generating a genuine moral dilemma.[9] According to Hindu thought, genuine dilemmas are paradoxical and are seldom solved. They may be resolved or dissolved, but not solved.

The concept of *dharma* can be useful in the examination of many of the moral dilemmas of the corporate executive, including the issue of the correctness of corporate decisions. As stated by Herbert A. Simon:

> Decisions are something more than factual proposition. To be sure, they are descriptive of a future state of affairs...but they possess, in addition, an imperative quality—they select one future state of affairs in preference to another and direct behavior toward the chosen alternative. In short, they have an ethical as well as a factual content.[10]

If genuine dilemmas are paradoxical and are seldom solved, what is the corporate executive to do? He or she has to be virtuous in decision making. The focus is on the obligations, and on the conflict between individual obligations and social responsibility. The goal has to be not so much to solve moral dilemmas as to *recognize* them.

An example would be helpful. There have been a number of instances where corporations have recalled products from the marketplace in the interests of the consumer and society. The recall of Tylenol by Johnson & Johnson or the Rely product by Procter and Gamble are examples of corporate decisions exhibiting uncommon virtue. In these instances, the executives decided on actions which did not necessarily fulfill their obligations to the stockholders, employees, and other parties. However, they acted to protect human welfare and save lives. They knew they faced a genuine moral dilemma. They did not solve the dilemma. They did not fulfill all their obligations. They opted to fulfill the obligation of social responsibility. They made this choice through enlightened wisdom, and they resolved the moral dilemma effectively.

The set of other familiar questions to which the concept of *dharma* could be applied for analysis include: What is the management's authority over corporate assets owned jointly by all stockholders? What is the validity of any act or transaction of the corporate executive? Is the corporate executive's preoccupation with playing the stock market akin to an addiction? When is gambling not gambling? Is the stock market similar to the gambling hall? What is the validity of any act fraudulently and deceitfully performed by cunning persons? Is corporate strategy, as we understand it, cunning? Is industrial espionage deceitful? What is the corporate executive's *dharma*? It would be helpful to examine further the concept of *dharma*.

What is Dharma?

According to Indian thought, *dharma* is one of the four major goals of human life, the others being *artha* (wealth), *kama* (enjoyment), and *moksa* (spiritual freedom). The term *dharma* is complex and has many meanings in the various Hindu writings. It deals with law and custom governing the development of individuals and with the proper relationships between different groups of society. In the context of this chapter, *dharma* refers to the basic principles of virtuous and righteous conduct. According to Manu, the author of *Manusmriti*, the term *dharma* includes the concepts of (1) law, usage, custom; (2) moral merit, virtue; (3) duty, prescribed code of conduct, obligation; (4) right, justice; (5) piety; (6) morality, ethics; (7) nature, character; and (8) an essential quality, characteristic property, an attribute.[11] With so many meanings to the word, the precise meaning of *dharma* is derived from the context of its usage. *Adharma* is the opposite of *dharma*, or devoid of *dharma*.

Professor K. Motwani of Jabalpur University has stated:

> *Dharma* is the cohesive element, and on the human plane, it is the principle of organization. From the standpoint of the individual, it is the implementing of the intellectual perception of his proper place and duties in the social cosmos; from the standpoint of the group, it is reason or intelligence...[that is] the basis of social life....It is here that the modernity of Manu's teachings comes in....[12]

Thus, Professor Motwani supports the earlier assertion that corporate executives must be able to recognize the conflict between individual obligations and social responsibiliies. The emphasis is clearly on the knowledge, or enlightened wisdom, required as a prerequisite to being virtuous.

In *Vaisheshika Sutra*, authored by Kanada after 300 B.C., *dharma* is described as a prerequisite for and cause of prosperity. According to the *vaisheshika* (particularity) system, *dharma* results in accomplishment of exaltation and the supreme good. *Dharma* is a property belonging to the person. It is particular, it depends to a large extent on the person's proper place and duties in the social system. "It is not a potency residing in the action performed." The *dharma* of the eldest brother relative to his younger brother is not entirely the same as that of the younger brother relative to his elder brother. The *dharma* of the *Brahman* (member of the priesthood) is different from that of the *Kshatriya* (member of the warrior class).

> The means of *dharma* consist of various substances, qualities and actions...some belonging in common to all men, and some as pertaining specially to distinct castes and conditions. Among the common ones we have the following: faith in *dharma*, harmlessness, benevolence, truthfulness, freedom from desire for undue possession, freedom from lust, purity of intentions, absence of anger, ...and non-neglect (of duties). *Dharma* is the direct cause of happiness, of the means of happiness and also of final deliverance ....*Dharma* is destructible....In as much as *dharma* is an effect, it must come to an end...it is an absolutely impartite entity....*Dharma* is also destroyed by true knowledge. Some people hold *dharma* to be absolutely indestructible; but for these people there could be no final deliverance; as there would be no end of *dharma* and *adharma* (and hence of the results of these in the shape of worldly experiences).

True knowledge leads people to become free from all affections, aversions and other such feelings. The absence of these sentiments causes cessation of *dharma* or *adharma*, tending toward "peace" and finally *moksa* (deliverance), emancipation, or liberation.[13]

Thus, it is *dharma* that leads to the behavior that promotes harmony in groups, in associations, in society and, indeed, in corporations; it facilitates growth and prosperity in all these. *Dharma* is related closely to *karma* (action or work), and *bhoga* (experience). This interconnection stands out clearly in the *Mahabharata*. We will examine now the "corporation problem" described in the *Mahabharata*, beginning with a description of the *Mahabharata* itself.

The Mahabharata

Sometime between 2000 and 1000 B.C., the Vedic scriptures were introduced into India, and gave the first framework to the Hindu religion. The period between 600 and 200 B.C. saw the emergence of philosophical doctrines through the medium of nontechnical literature, specially the great epics, the *Ramayana* and the *Mahabharata* (including the *Bhagavad-Gita* which is a part of the *Mahabharata*). This period includes the rise and early development of Buddhism, Vaishnavism, Shaivism and Jainism. It was during this period also that many of the *Dharmashastras*, or treatises on ethical and social philosophy, describing the ethical and religious obligations of the Aryans, were compiled. *Manusmriti* (the *Code of Manu*) was one such treatise. The *Mahabharata* is a *kavya* (an epic poem), a *Dharmashashtra* (a treatise on ethics and righteous conduct), and an *Itihasa* (a book of history). It discloses a rich civilization in a highly evolved society. India was divided into a number of independent kingdoms, yet there was a unified concept of culture and *dharma*. There was an accepted code of warfare, deviations from which were met with reproof among *Kshatriyas*. The population lived in cities and villages. There was trade in the cities, and the mass of people were agriculturists. In addition to urban and rural life, there was a highly cultured life in the seclusion of forests "ashrams," presided over by respected and revered ascetic teachers. The caste system prevailed but inter-caste marriages did take place and Brahmans did take arms in war. Women were honored and played important roles in the lives of their husbands and children. As stated before, and as we shall see, in the *Mahabharata* the "corporation problem" is described in the context of "a husband's supremacy over his wife" or the lack thereof. It would be helpful, therefore, to review briefly the status of women in that culture.

The Status of Women

According to the *Manusmriti*, women are precious, to be "honoured and adorned" by their fathers, brothers, husbands and brothers-in-law who desire welfare. Life and the continued existence of family and the society depend on women. "Where women are honoured, there the gods are pleased....Where the female relations live in grief, the family soon wholly perishes; but that family where they are not unhappy ever prospers." A woman usually is physically weaker than a man and in possession of qualities which make her likely to be forcibly usurped by other persons even against her wish. For this reason, she is to be protected at all times, by her father in her childhood, husband in her adulthood, and son in her old age:

> By a girl, by a young woman, or even by an aged one, nothing must be done independently, even in her own house....In childhood a female must be subject to her father, in youth to her husband, when [he] is dead to her sons; a woman must never be independent.[14]

Dyuta: A Game of Chance

The *Mahabharata* gives an account of the feud between two families, the Kauravas and the Pandavas, both of whose ancestries could be traced to Vichitravirya and Santanu. The Kaurava family was large and included Duryodhana, Karna, Bhishma, Duhshashna, Vikarna and many others. The Pandavas consisted of five brothers—Yudhishthira, Nakula, Sahadeva, Arjuna and Bhimsena; all five were husbands to Draupadi, daughter of Drupada, King of the Panchalas. The account of Draupadi's marriage to the five Pandava brothers is the sole instance of polyandrous marriage in the *Mahabharata*.

The first event of the series that resulted in the carnage at the battle-field of Kurukshetra was a gambling match into which Yudhishthira, the Pandava emperor, was trapped by Sakuni, the evil genius and advisor to Duryodhana. Sakuni's goal was to assist Duryodhana in acquiring Yudhishthira's kingdom. At Sakuni's insistence, Duryodhana persuaded his father Dhritarashtra, the blind Kaurava king, to invite Yudhishthira to *dyuta* (a game of dice). Even though Dhritarashtra protested, "Your suggestion does not seem proper," being weak-witted and over-persuaded, he yielded to his son's desire. Yudhishthira, on receiving the invitation through Vidura, Dhritarashtra's chief counselor and emissary, responded, "O King! gambling is bad. It is not through heroism or merit that one succeeds in a game of chance. Asita, Devala and other wise *rishis* who were well versed in worldly affairs have declared that gambling should be avoided since it offers scope for deceit. They have also said that conquest in battle is the proper path for the *Kshatriyas*."[15] Yet Yudhishthira was fond of gambling and the *Kshatriya* tradition made it a matter of etiquette and honor not to refuse an invitation to a game of dice. On an earlier occasion, Sage Vyasa had warned Yudhishthira of the quarrels to come between the two families, leading to the destruction of their race.

Yudhishthira had promised Vyasa that he would not give the Kauravas cause for displeasure. Yudhishthira accepted the invitation and, with his Pandava brothers, arrived in the Kaurava capital of Hastinapura.

When *dyuta* began, Yudhishthira played against Sakuni. At first they wagered jewels, gold and silver, then chariots and horses. Yudhishthira lost continuously, and Sakuni played tricks. Stakes increased. Yudhishthira lost cities, villages, his brothers' ornaments and his own, as well as the clothes they wore. Yudhishthira's response to the unbroken string of losses was a stubborn commitment to the game. He wagered his brothers. He lost them, one by one. They became Kaurava slaves. Then he wagered himself and lost.

When it was clear that Sakuni had won Yudhishthira, thus making him a slave as well, he said to Yudhishthira, "O King! That you lost yourself is no good; because losing oneself is a sin when some wealth is left there." It must be noted that Sakuni acknowledged that Yudhishthira had lost himself. He even announced to all the kings present in the gambling hall that the Pandavas had been lost. Then Sakuni said to Yudhishthira, "O King! There is one jewel still in your possession by staking which you can yet free yourself. Can you not continue the game offering your wife Draupadi as wager?"[16] Here again, Sakuni acknowledged that Yudhishthira had been conquered. Yudhishthira staked Draupadi. There were cries of "Shame! Shame!" from spectators, but none prevented Yudhishthira from betting Draupadi in this manner. Sakuni won this round as well. Duryodhana ordered Vidura to fetch Draupadi and to bring her to the Kaurava *sabha* (assembly). It was his contention that Draupadi, having been lost by Yudhishthira, was henceforth a Kaurava *dasi* (slave) and he announced that Draupadi from then on would "sweep and clean our house." Vidura refused to do so. He turned to the assembly and said, "Yudhishthira had no right to stake Draupadi as by then he had himself already lost his freedom and lost all rights." According to Vidura, Draupadi could not become a slave because Yudhishthira had no authority to bet her, having lost himself to Sakuni. Thus, Vidura was the first in the *Mahabharata* to raise the issue of "the corporation problem" by pointing to the separation of ownership and control. It is not clear whether Sakuni had recognized this subtle point. He had acknowledged repeatedly that Yudhishthira had lost his independence, but had never alluded to the complications that followed.

Duryodhana rebuked the virtuous and wise Vidura, and sent his own charioteer, Prathikami, to bring Draupadi to the assembly. Draupadi was dumbfounded at the strange message conveyed to her by the charioteer. "Which prince would pledge his wife?" she asked, "Had he nothing else to pawn?" Prathikami narrated how Yudhishthira already had lost all his possessions, his brothers and himself, and then her. Draupadi asked Prathikami to return to the Kaurava assembly and "Ask of him who played the game whether in it he first lost himself, or his wife." She added, "Ask this question in the open assembly; bring me his answer and then you can take me." [17] The issue of the separation of ownership and control was not lost on Draupadi. Ultimately, Draupadi was dragged to the assembly by Duhshashna. Again she asked whether the members of the assembly thought that, according to law, she was enslaved.

The situation greatly troubled the wise, virtuous and righteous Bhishma. He spoke thus: "*Dharma* being subtle, I cannot quite properly analyze your question; no one who is not master can stake another's wealth; but a wife is always under the supremacy of her husband." Bhishma thus indicated that Yudhishthira had lost authority over Draupadi by first losing himself and, therefore, could not bet her. He indicated also that a husband's authority over his wife was never lost. Therefore, Bhishma admitted that he was unable to answer Draupadi's question.[18]

Bhishma made another point. He told Draupadi that Sakuni was an expert in the game of dice, and had induced Yudhishthira to put her at stake. He noted that Yudhishthira never gave up *dharma* nor accused Sakuni of deceit, "Hence I cannot answer your question." The point is that if one is induced fraudulently to act in a particular way, then that transaction becomes invalid. However, the complaint must come from the person affected. Yudhishthira probably did not complain for the same reasons that impelled him to accept the invitation to the *dyuta* in the first place.

Draupadi stressed the fraudulent nature of the transaction and its invalidity. She accused the fraudulent and cunning gamblers, expert in the game of dice, of impure intentions. She accused them of cheating and asked the assembly to state clearly and properly why Yudhishthira was induced to play a game of dice? No one answered. Duryodhana's brother, Vikarna, was astonished to see his elders, Dhritarashtra, Bhishma, Dronacharya and others who were known for their judgment and wisdom, unable to restrain Duryodhana. Finally, he rose and made this statement: "O *Kshatriya* heroes, why are you silent? I am a mere youth,

I know, but your silence compels me to speak." Vikarna first pointed out that Yudhishthira was enticed to this game by a deeply plotted invitation. This invitation took advantage of Yudhishthira's weakness for the vice of gambling. He pointed out that Draupadi was wife to all five Pandavas; therefore, Yudhishthira had pledged Draupadi when he had no right to do so because she did not belong only to him. For that reason alone, Vikarna asserted, the wager was illegal. Besides, Yudhishthira already had lost his freedom and, therefore, had no right to offer her as a stake. Vikarna continued, "And there is this further objection. It was Sakuni who suggested [Draupadi] as a pledge, which is against the rules of the game, under which neither player must demand a specific bet. If we consider all these points, we must admit that Draupadi has not been legally won by us. This is my opinion."

After Vikarna's speech, Duryodhana said to Draupadi that if all other four Pandavas stated clearly that Yudhishthira had no authority to put Draupadi as a bet, she would be freed. Bhimsena spoke, but did not meet Duryodhana's condition. Others kept quiet. When Duryodhana repeated his offer, Arjuna said that Yudhishthira had full authority to put each brother at stake before he lost himself. But when he himself was conquered, he could not bet Draupadi. At this point there were some ugly scenes in the gambling hall, and Dhritarashtra intervened at last. He stopped all further proceedings, chided Duryodhana and, with due sympathy and respect, granted boons to Draupadi. She asked for the release of Yudhishthira from bondage, and secured the release of the other four Pandavas. Dhritarashtra then ordered the return of all wealth and the kingdom to Yudhishthira. The Pandavas returned to Indraprastha with full honor and authority. Here the first *dyuta* ended. Another one was to follow but that is not the concern of this chapter.

Discussion

Now let us discuss the main problems emerging from the *dyuta* described above. Such discussion will provide insights as to how the concept of *dharma* was applied by the various characters in the first *dyuta* incident of the *Mahabharata*. Vidura pointed out that Yudhishthira had lost himself first and so had no further authority to bet Draupadi. Bhishma and Arjuna also considered this to be a valid point, although Bhishma seemed confounded by the consideration of a husband's supremacy over a wife. Bhishma was inclined to think that a husband's supremacy over his wife remained unchanged. This principle implied that the supremacy of the other four Pandavas over Draupadi also remained unchanged. But Bhishma did not take his analysis that far. If he had, he would have had to have concluded that Draupadi could not be bet unilaterally by Yudhishthira. Another line of argument could be pursued: The four Pandava brothers did not object to Yudhishthira's staking them at the *dyuta*. This implies that the Pandava brothers accepted Yudhishthira's supremacy over them as the eldest brother. This, in fact, was consistent with their *dharma*. One's eldest brother was to be held in the same regard as one's father. The four Pandava brothers also did not object to Yudhishthira's staking Draupadi at the *dyuta*. If, like Bhishma, they believed that a husband's supremacy over his wife remained unchanged, they would have indicated this when Yudhishthira staked Draupadi (unless they regarded Yudhishthira's supremacy over them as superseding theirs over Draupadi). Perhaps, having been enslaved themselves they saw themselves as having lost supremacy over Draupadi and, therefore, Yudhishthira's supremacy over them remained intact.

Vikarna supported the view that Yudhishthira could not exercise unilateral supremacy over Draupadi because she was wife to all Pandavas. Since all Pandavas had been enslaved before Draupadi was staked, Vikarna rejected the notion that Draupadi had been enslaved. However, the Pandavas did not press this issue and accepted the authority of Yudhishthira; therefore, this point could not be tested. The argument that a fraudulent and deceitful transaction is invalid is a persuasive one but, here too, Yudhishthira did not press this issue nor complain.[19]

Draupadi, it appears, did not consider herself to be enslaved. She had asked the assembly to give its verdict as to whether or not she had been enslaved, but received no answer. However, when Dhritarashtra bestowed boons upon her, she asked for the freedom of the Pandavas; she did not ask for her own freedom, which suggests that she did not consider herself enslaved because Yudhishthira had lost authority over her as her husband after he lost himself to Sakuni.

Vikarna raised another interesting issue concerning the validity of an addict's act. According to Vikarna, Draupadi did not constitute a valid stake because Yudhishthira was engrossed in gambling at the time. This argument does not hold well because Yudhishthira rightly could not be regarded as an addict. Finally, there is the question of authority of the husband over his wife; does it cease in certain circumstances or is it limitless? Only Bhishma considered this point but he did not express a clear opinion. Others did not discuss this issue explicitly either; however, it can be inferred that they considered that the husband's authority was not limitless—it ceased under certain circumstances.

As stated, in Hindu thought genuine dilemmas are regarded as unsolvable. Bhishma and Duryodhana make for an interesting contrast in character. They were Kaurava brothers, yet Bhishma was committed to *dharma* and experienced anguish at the plight of the Pandava brothers. He told Yudhishthira that man is the slave of wealth, whereas wealth has no slave. He said he was bound to the Kaurava's wealth and, therefore, felt helpless about Yudhishthira's plight even though he believed the Pandavas were just. Thus he requested that Yudhishthira excuse him from taking a stand, and Yudhishthira complied, freeing Bhishma from his dilemma. Duryodhana, on the other hand, lacking virtue, devoid of *dharma* and practicing *adharma,* was blinded by greed and hatred for the Pandavas; he experienced no moral dilemma.

In the context of corporate ownership and control, three points of consideration are suggested by the above:

(1) What is the nature of management's authority over corporate assets owned jointly by all stockholders?
(2) What is the validity of any act or transaction of an addict (irrespective of evidence of addiction or its absence in this case)?
(3) What is the validity of any act fraudulently and deceitfully performed by cunning persons?

Yudhishthira, on receiving the invitation through Vidura, had responded by stating that gambling was bad because dice was a game of chance and, therefore, it was not through merit that one succeeded; success was accidental.

Would the modern-day financial system, centered around Wall Street, be a game of chance? And what of the issue raised earlier regarding addiction? Yudhishthira was accused of being addicted to gambling. Modern corporations are "addicted" to the financial markets, as evidenced by the importance of stock exchanges all over the world. When is gambling not gambling any more but a prudent, even virtuous, act? And, of course, is industrial espionage and corporate strategy cunning and deceitful? Is it appropriate for a corporation to raid other corporations for scientists, strategists and employees to learn about their firm's strategies and plans? Would such actions be consistent with the corporate executive's *dharma*?

Conclusion

The concept of *dharma* does not insist on solving a moral dilemma. It does, however, insist and expects that the individual *recognize* a moral dilemma when confronted with one, which is why Bhishma is regarded as superior to Duryodhana. Bhishma recognized his dilemma and its subtlety. Duryodhana was oblivious to his own dilemma and so acted irresponsibly. The focus of the corporate executive's *dharma* is on the conflict between individual duty and social responsibility. Virtue is a necessary prerequisite for moral choice. And enlightenment is necessary for virtue.

Notes

1. A.D. Chandler, *Strategy and Structure: Chapters in the History of the Industrial Enterprise* (Cambridge, MA: Massachusetts Institute of Technology Press, 1962).

2. J. Greenwald, "Predator's Fall," *Time*, February 26, 1990, pp. 46-52.

3. H.E. Krooss and C. Gilbert, *American Business History* (Englewood Cliffs, NJ: Prentice-Hall, Inc., 1972), p. 264.

4. *Ibid.*, p. 247.

5. Greenwald, pp. 47-48.

6. M. Weber, *Wirtschaft und Gesellschaft: Grundriss der Verstehen Soziologie* (Cologne: Kiepenheuer and Witsch, 1964), p. l:366.

7. I. Kant, *The Metaphysics of Morals, 1*, trans. J. Ladd (Indianapolis, IN: Bobbs-Merrill, 1965) in *Moral Dilemmas in the Mahabharata*, ed. B.K. Matilal (Shimla, India: Indian Institute of Advanced Study, 1989), p. 8.

8. R.B. Marcus, "Moral Dilemma and Consistency." *Journal of Philosophy*, 77, 1980, pp. 121-136.

9. B.K. Matilal, "Moral Dilemmas: Insights from Indian Epics," *Moral Dilemmas in the Mahabharata*, pp. 8-9.

10. H.A. Simon, *Administrative Behavior*, Second Edition (New York, NY: The Free Press, 1965). p. 46.

11. M.V. Patwardhan, *Manusmriti: The Ideal Democratic Republic of Manu* (Delhi, India: Motilal Banarsidass, 1968), p. 80.

12. *Ibid.*, p. vii.

13. S. Radhakrishnan and C.A. Moore, eds., *A Source Book in Indian Philosophy*, Second Edition (Princeton, NJ: Princeton University Press, 1960), pp. 416-418.

14. *Ibid.*, pp. 189-192.

15. C. Rajagopalachari, *Mahabharata*, Eighth Edition (Bombay, India: Bharatiya Vidya Bhavan, 1966), pp. 87-88.

16. *Ibid.*, p. 90.

17. *Ibid.*, p. 91.

18. S.M. Kulkarni, "An Unresolved Dilemma in *Dyuta-parvan*: A Question Raised by Draupadi," *Moral Dilemmas in the Mahabharata* (Shimla, India: Indian Institute of Advanced Study, 1989), p. 152.

19. *Ibid.*, p. 154.

Part II

Business Stories:
Do They Make a Difference?

Maturity of judgment involves the rational capacity to see all the issues, to sort out the gut issues from the peripheral ones, the ones in need of prompt solution from those permitting or requiring a longer period for resolution, and so forth. As to qualities of moral character, I believe the essential ingredient is the capacity for empathy, the ability to put oneself in the place of those persons with whom one is dealing or those persons who will be affected by a decision. Many, if not most, of the people I know who have achieved a high degree of competence in their chosen areas have such ego problems, or are so insensitive to what is going on in the minds and hearts of other parties, that despite their competence they have no capacity for judgment in situations where the ability to foresee consequences counts for a great deal. After all, the most difficult part of foresight is that of anticipating likely actions on the part of other free agents who will be reacting to one's judgment. If one is so insensitive or so self-absorbed that he cannot put himself in the other person's position, then he will be quite a limited person.

Elmer W. Johnson

Churches have been, and ought to be, communities of moral formation. But this is not always the case, for many reasons. One has to think carefully both about how morals are formed, and about what values and principles and ideals are to be fostered. Your "effective" person really exercises agency; a religious moral nurture around rigid rules would not fully prepare a person to be a responsive agent. Churches are failing as communities of moral nurture or formation....

James M. Gustafson

A distinguished corporate executive who has served also in government visited Stanford Business School and was asked what the similarities were between his top management experience in business and government. In both jobs, he reported, he was called on continually to make difficult trade-offs between two or more stakeholders, or between a petitioner and a proper concept of the public interest. "I've concluded," he said, "that the manager is best described as a practicing ethicist."

Kirk O. Hanson

Defining business ethics is far from simple, but it is not impossible. The wisest observers of the investment community will approach this topic with humility. Imagining that we can define and codify business ethics in a precise, neat list of commands would be as dangerous a mistake as thinking we can define ethical conduct as mere adherence to the law.

John J. Phelan, Jr.

• • • • •

Two observers of the morality of large organizations, Michael Bowen and Clark Power, detail the lengthy story of a wreck that has been much in the news of late:

> Since March 24, 1989, when the supertanker *Exxon Valdez* ran aground on Alaska's Bligh Reef spilling some 240,000 barrels (about 11 million gallons or 170,000 tons) of crude oil into the surrounding waters of Prince William Sound, countless questions have been asked as to why the disaster occurred, where to put the blame, and how such spills can be prevented. Although there has been a great deal of retrospective analysis, solutions to these problems appear to be attached to the self-interests of the constituents providing the "answers." Corrective policy decisions thus are awash in claims and counter-claims, lawsuits and counter-lawsuits, and debates that pit expert against expert. It would seem that every constituent involved not only has a favorite scapegoat but also a set of "should's" that would solve the problems of safely delivering the rich Alaskan crude oil to a energy-hungry America.

The business ethicist, John Houck, reflects on a story from the pages of the *Wall Street Journal:*

> For instance, supposing our manager was using an image in his
> life which was consciously biblical. Could it set the context for
> his deliberations about the plant closing? He might see himself,
> based on religious conviction, as a Servant, which would mean
> he sees himself as a person *and* a manager, *thrust into the hopes
> and ambitions of the world, and yet having a calling to realize God's
> love and justice.* The Jesus Story, here interpreted as a model of
> one who came to serve and *not* to be served, can affect and even
> change our manager's perception of self and personal ambition.
> It can also change the business world about him.
>
> Our manager, because of his appropriation of the Servant
> Image, wants to save the jobs in the New England town.
> Therefore, he can be described as a person of good will, but he
> must have the co-requisite competence to save the jobs.

Dennis McCann, professor of religious studies and co-director of the
Center for the Study of Values at DePaul University, writes:

> I will argue that business people do not need to be sold on a
> narrative approach to understanding morality, for storytelling is
> clearly the preferred way by which individuals are socialized into
> the ethos of business as a whole as well as into particular
> corporate cultures. What is called for, therefore, is not another
> apology for narrative but a critical evaluation of the stories
> already communicated in the world of business. If this story line
> is still capable of communicating an authentically Christian
> vision of the world in which we work out our salvation, it must
> be as capable of being discerned in the stories of business people
> and institutions as it is in any other walk of life.

The legal ethicist, Thomas Shaffer, writes about the state of business
stories in our culture:

> But it is unusual to find a story about someone who is a good
> person, in business, in the U.S. Our culture, which has produced
> more sustained business success than any other, and which has
> distributed the benefits of business more widely than any other,

has produced almost no business hero stories. If you consult only our stories you will decide that our business people are self-deceived or rapacious, or both. Which means something is skewed. The value of stories in ethics is that they give access to common sense with relatively little interference from concepts. Common sense says that business in the U.S. is not corrupting, even if business stories say it is. We know good people in business. Some of them are in *big* business. They live next door to us; we worship with them; we get wise advice from them as we buy our cough medicine and hardware. They are our parents and our children, our sisters, brothers, aunts and uncles. They are our friends, and friendship, Aristotle says, is collaboration in the good....The problem, I suspect, is that our popular stories about business are not in touch with reality.

Six

Exxon's Knee-Deep in the Big Muddy*

A Case Study of Managerial Ethics, Decisions, and Decision Making, Based on Circumstances Surrounding the 1989 Exxon Valdez Oil Spill

Michael G. Bowen and F. Clark Power

Since March 24, 1989, when the supertanker *Exxon Valdez* ran aground on Alaska's Bligh Reef spilling some 240,000 barrels (about 11 million gallons or 170,000 tons) of crude oil into the surrounding waters of Prince William Sound, countless questions have been asked as to why the disaster occurred, where to put the blame, and how such spills can be prevented. Although there has been a great deal of retrospective analysis, solutions to these problems appear to be attached to the self-interests of the constituents providing the "answers." Corrective policy decisions thus are awash in claims and counter-claims, lawsuits and counter-lawsuits, and dabates that pit expert against expert. It would seem that every constituent involved not only has a favorite scapegoat but also a set of "should's" that would solve the problems of safely delivering the rich Alaskan crude oil to a energy-hungry America.

Clearly, however, the Exxon Corporation and the captain of the *Exxon Valdez*, Joseph Hazelwood, have taken the brunt of the blame for the tragedy. Even after acknowledging responsibility shortly after the accident and promising that the spill would be cleaned up, Exxon—in particular its top executives, Chairman Lawrence G. Rawl and President Lee Raymond—has been the subject of many harsh criticisms that include criminal indictments and calls for the chairman's resignation. One result of this has been great damage to Exxon's carefully cultivated reputation as one of the world's most esteemed corporations.

*Permission granted by the Ethics in Business Program, Graduate School of Business, Columbia University, New York.

What is there to learn from this case? Is there a simple solution to be found, one that was "there all the time" and that would have prevented the spill? Is one course of action "right" and others "wrong"? How would one manage Exxon so that shareholders, employees, environmentalists, the various governments involved, and other company constituencies *all* remain satisfied over time? Is there a set of actions to identify the "perfect" management of the Exxon Corporation? If so, what would these actions be and how would they affect those who manage the trade-offs among a business organization's competitive, organizational, fiduciary, legal, and ethics/moral responsibilities on an ongoing basis?

To encourage a realistic consideration of these issues we have broken this case into four sections, each representing a different portion of the events surrounding the spill: (1) the pre-accident period; (2) the time of the accident; (3) the cleanup period; and (4) the post-cleanup period. These situations, although certainly related, present unique management questions and challenges.

The Pre-Accident Period

On Friday, March 13, 1968, a field containing an estimated 10 billion barrels of oil was discovered under the North Slope of Alaska at Prudhoe Bay. One year later, a consortium of seven oil companies, now named the Alyeska Pipeline Service Company, announced plans to construct an 800-mile-long underground pipeline to some point in southern Alaska where the crude oil could be transferred to tankers and shipped to refineries in the lower 48 states. The eventual choice for the oil terminal was an ice-free port, tucked away in the Chugach Mountains on the northern banks of Prince William Sound, that provided easy access to the Gulf of Alaska and shipping lanes to California: the town of Valdez.

The oil companies' original plans called for construction to begin on the trans-Alaskan pipeline in the following year (1970). They projected that the pipeline would be completed two years later. Approximately 2 million barrels of oil per day would be pumped from stations on the North Slope to Valdez Harbor where tankers would carry the oil south. The companies, however, had not counted on the powerful reaction of environmental interest groups to their plans.

Over the next four years the environmental and economic effects of the proposed pipeline were subject to intense scrutiny. There was little substantive disagreement on the purely economic issues: The oil companies, the state of Alaska, and many Alaskans would make a great deal of money if the pipeline were built. Many other benefits would result directly from the pipeline project. Of these, perhaps the most important was the development of a major new domestic source of oil reserves which would reduce the United States' dependency on foreign energy sources. There was also surprisingly little disagreement on the environmental issues. The oil companies admitted that there was the possibility of accidents and spills, perhaps major ones. There was agreement that the permafrost along the pipeline would melt, that wildlife would be affected adversely, and that portions of Alaska's wilderness and extraordinary scenery would be either defaced or destroyed.

There was substantial disagreement, however, on how to estimate the benefits and costs that would accrue from shipping oil across Alaska. How should the tangible benefits of economic development in the region be weighed against the intangible costs of defacing Alaska's pristine scenery; of disturbing the habitat of the vanishing bald eagles, bears and caribou; of poisoning fish and damaging the food chain?

However, the trans-Alaskan pipeline was approved in 1973 when the U.S. Congress, reacting to the possibility of fuel shortages in this country and to the repeated assurances of oil industry and government experts that policies and procedures would be put in place to meet environmental contingencies, cut off the court challenges that had delayed construction. At a U.S. Department of the Interior hearing held in Anchorage in 1971, for example, Alyeska representatives pledged that the environmental effects of the pipeline operations would be minimal, promising prompt and effective handling of any land or sea spill. They announced that an oil response plan would be prepared so that operations at the Port of Valdez and in Prince William Sound would be the safest in the world. While the Alyeska consortium would shoulder responsibility to clean up any spills, the task of monitoring Alyeska's preparedness would be handled by the Coast Guard and the state of Alaska. Behind the scenes, Alyeska officials recognized (as can be documented in their actual cleanup plan) that it would be impossible for them to clean up a major spill.

Only Once in 241 Years

For the first couple of years after oil began flowing through the pipeline in 1977, Alyeska's performance at responding to oil spills, as reported by state of Alaska officials, was excellent. Detailed records were kept on the cleanup of even very minor spills, such as crankcase oil dripping underneath a parked automobile. No doubt part of this vigilance was due to the 1978 sinking of the supertanker *Amoco Cadiz* off the coast of France, which resulted in a spill six times larger than that of the *Exxon Valdez*.

Alyeska's safety record for the remainder of the first decade of the pipeline's operation continued to be strong. Although 25 percent of the oil pumped from the ground in the United States passes through the Port of Valdez, by the end of 1988, 400 reported spills had leaked only about 200 barrels into the Alaskan waters. In the three-month period from November 1988 through January 1989, however, 43 spills were reported in Alaskan waters—ranging in size from 10,000 to 2 million gallons— including a 1,700 barrel leak (efficiently contained and cleaned up) from a tanker docked at the Valdez terminal. In spite of this increase in accidents, Alyeska officials still seemed content that a major spill was not a realistic possibility. Why were they so complacent?

In the first place, the basis for Alyeska's contingency planning, an independent report conducted for the oil company consortium and approved by the state, concluded that a spill of between 1,000-2,000 barrels (46,000-92,000 gallons) was the most likely disaster that could occur in the projected 30-year lifetime of the Valdez terminal. Because the route from Valdez Harbor to the Gulf of Alaska was relatively easy to navigate, and because of the safeguards to be put in place before shipping began, a catastrophic spill like that of the *Exxon Valdez* was thought to be extremely unlikely—only once in 241 years. Nevertheless, when it was time for Alyeska and the state to negotiate a new 3-year contingency plan, the state requested that Alyeska develop a scenario for dealing with a major spill. Alyeska officals balked, as they had whenever regulatory demands had been made. The compromise left Alyeska geared up to contain and clean up spills almost 175 times smaller than the *Exxon Valdez* spill.

Why did the state of Alaska ever agree to such a plan? What had happened to the oversight the state and the Coast Guard had promised? From the moment the pipeline opened, the people of Alaska have benefitted from the approximately $400,000 per hour in state revenues that have accrued. In the ensuing years, as the state became more and more financially dependent on oil monies and as no major spill had occurred, vigilance over the pipeline operation slowly began to relax.

Warnings?

The first warnings concerning the deterioration of state monitoring and Alyeska's ill-preparedness came in 1983 from Dan Lawn, Alaska's Department of Environmental Conservation (DEC) inspector who detailed his charges in a 1984 memo. For all practical purposes they were ignored. In 1984 Alyeska failed to contain a relatively small (60 barrel) simulated loading spill in a state-administered test of the consortium's response capability. In 1986 Lawn judged that Alyeska failed again, although other judges rated Alyeska's performance as marginally passable. As Lawn became more critical, Alyeska officials resorted to calling him a "jerk and a trouble maker," and George Nelson, the president, admits trying to get Lawn fired. Lawn persisted in his warnings, predicting only three months before the Valdez incident that the odds favored a major spill and no one would be prepared.

Why was no one listening, especially at the state and federal levels? Three reasons appear obvious. First, the collapse of oil prices between 1984 and 1985 reduced the state's oil income from over $4 billion to under $2 billion per year. Alaska, which generated over 80 percent of its revenues from oil, was forced to cut services. Subsequently, the agency charged with monitoring Alyeska and the operations at the Valdez terminal, the DEC, cut staff to the point where there was no full-time state monitor of the oil terminal operations.

Second, the relative absence of serious trouble seemed to justify reductions in preparedness. With the safe passage of so many vessels through the Sound, the Coast Guard came to believe it could reduce its inspections of tankers coming into and leaving Valdez Harbor. Over time, staffing of the Coast Guard monitoring station was cut back, around-the-clock supervision at the radar console was eliminated and, to reduce paperwork, the Coast Guard in 1987 stopped manual plotting of ships' courses in and out of the channel. Further, the Coast Guard also judged proposals for an advanced radar system and an additional navigation monitoring system that would have tracked tanker traffic through the channel more effectively (and would have included a radar site on Bligh Island) to be too costly for the value added.

Third, as public attention shifted to other environmental concerns, pressure to develop technology to prevent and clean up low-probability spills eased. For example, the federal government decided in 1987 to shut down the Oil and Hazardous Material Simulated Environmental Test Tank (OHMSETT) research facility in New Jersey.

Exxon

The relatively sudden, drastic drop in oil prices also hit the companies hard. In contrast to foreign competitors, the domestic companies in the industry were under pressure from the U.S. investment community to become more productive and efficient. Therefore, they had to curtail what could be identified as "unnecessary" expenditures within their organizations so that profitability would be stabilized at an acceptable level. Precautionary measures such as putting double hulls around tankers, effectively reducing cargo area by 25 percent and dramatically increasing the cost of oil vessels, were ruled out as being not cost-effective.

Unlike many of its competitors in the oil industry that had resorted to heavy cost cutting and organizational restructurings in the early to mid-1980s, the Exxon Corporation initially turned to a diversification strategy to bolster sagging performance. During this time, Exxon invested heavily in non-oil ventures such as office automation and electrical equipment, both later proving to be costly failures. More drastic internal changes began at Exxon in late 1986, only a few months before Lawrence Rawl, a long-time Exxon employee who was described by co-workers as blunt and arrogant, became chairman. Armed with a reputation as a heavy handed "cost-cutter," Rawl directed Exxon's down-sizing. As a result, within two years, company employment fell 30 percent to around 100,000 as he eliminated layers of bureaucracy, consolidated operations, and sold off unprofitable businesses.

Efforts to become more productive at Exxon during this time often meant large changes in the way the company did business and worked with employees. In addition to layoffs, reassignments and job restructurings, Exxon implemented any technological improvements which would lower its cost of doing business. This led to, among other things, taking the industry lead in constructing new, more highly automated oil tankers, for example, the *Exxon Valdez,* that could function with smaller crews.

To implement plans for higher efficiency within the company, managers were given some latitude in devising the desired productivity improvements. Some embraced the ideas of noted management expert W. Edwards Deming. The chief importer of modern Japanese management techniques, Deming stresses commitment to change, continuous innovation and quality improvement, and removal of communication barriers between workers and supervisors. At the same time, however, other managers subscribed to the Japanese practice of finding and achieving maximum productivity through pushing work systems to their productive limits, i.e., to the point where they start to crack and workers can no longer handle the load. While implementing these changes, management discovered, as have many companies that have been put through similar restructurings, that predictable problems arose: serious complaints of overwork, an erosion of management confidence, and sagging morale. "The problem with restructuring," Rawl has said since, "is the human factor: Can people perform the job they're given? You can't test a person like a computer chip."

The changes made at the Exxon Corporation in those days did, however, seem to "work" for the company's shareholders. In 1987, for example, the leaner and meaner Exxon netted $375 million more than it had the previous year. The corporation earned a net profit of $48,400 per employee in 1987, more than double the profit of key competitor Amoco and five times more than Mobil during the same period.

March 23, 1989

On Thursday night, March 23, 1989, no one was particularly worried about the *Exxon Valdez* or any of the other tankers slowly being filled with rich North Slope Alaskan crude oil in Valdez Harbor. The state of Alaska was depressed still but recovering from its deepest financial woes, yet it had not deemed it necessary to expand its vigilance of oil operations there. Perhaps no one from the DEC knew about or was concerned with the fact that Alyeska's single oil spill emergency barge was in dry dock for repairs.

There was nothing out of the ordinary going on in Prince William Sound that evening, not even the free floating icebergs drifting through the waters of the Sound. As had become the routine time-saving practice, Hazelwood steered around the icebergs rather than slowing down and staying in his traffic lane (the safer procedure). For members of the U.S. Coast Guard on duty in Valdez, this was just another quiet night—a night just like all the other nights since the port was opened to oil traffic twelve years earlier.

For the leaders of the Exxon Corporation, this also seemed like just another quiet evening. Rawl spent the evening at home. For Hazelwood and his shipmates, it had been just another exhausting day. Having put in long hours (the usual double duty) as the ship was loading, the crew was very tired. Even so, the captain of the *Exxon Valdez* and two of his mates stopped by a local tavern for a few drinks. At 9:25 that Thursday evening the supertanker left the terminal at Valdez Harbor, loaded with 1,250,000 barrels of crude oil.

At the Time of the Accident

Four minutes after midnight on March 24, 1989, about two and one-half hours into their journey south with an inexperienced third mate in command, the crew of the *Exxon Valdez* felt a sudden jolt and the ship begin to shudder, a sickening shudder that lasted about ten seconds. Eventually more than 240,000 barrels, or about 11 million gallons, of crude oil would gush into the surrounding waters. Hazelwood later said, "I knew we'd struck something; something major had happened to the vessel. I didn't know, but over the years you feel different things. I'd had engines blow up, other groundings, but it's an unhealthy feeling."

Afterward, Hazelwood recalled his feelings, "You don't know if you want to cry, throw up, or scream all at the same time; knowing at the same time you've got a job to do." Despite these mixed feelings, or perhaps because of them, the captain rushed to the ship's bridge from his quarters below, and went to work. With the supertanker listing on its right side— oil gushing from a 600-foot tear in its hull—and apparently balancing precariously on a narrow ledge, Chief Mate James Kunkel told the captain that he feared for all of their lives, and that he thought the supertanker would capsize if it came off the reef.

At 12:26 a.m., 22 minutes after striking the reef, Hazelwood (as he tells it: "trying not to cry, and [trying to] be reasonably businesslike") matter-of-factly radioed the Coast Guard station at Valdez. He was to be criticized later by the state of Alaska for being so calm in his radio transmissions. In Valdez, the Coast Guard watchperson who took the call put down his paperwork, adjusted the radar so the *Exxon Valdez* came into view, and confirmed that the supertanker was indeed aground on Bligh Reef. Several minutes later, the superintendent of operations at Alyeska's Valdez terminal was awakened with news of the accident. Following the "book" on such incidents, he told a subordinate to take charge and went back to sleep. When Coast Guard Vice Admiral Clyde Robbins was informed about the grounding he responded, "That's impossible. We have the perfect system." As he watched the oil from his ship pouring into the water, Hazelwood thought, "My world as I had known it had come to an end. "

At approximately 12:49 a.m. Hazelwood radioed the Coast Guard that, despite having a little trouble with the third mate and the fact that the ship had been "holed," he was trying to get the ship off the reef and would get back in touch as soon as he could.

Exxon's Response

At 8:30 a.m. that day (4:30 a.m. Valdez time), the kitchen phone rang as Rawl was having breakfast in his Westchester County, N.Y., home. He remembers asking the caller what had happened, if a rudder had broken, and if the ship had lost its engine. "At that point I didn't even know what it hit. All I knew was that it hit something and it was holed pretty badly," Rawl is quoted as saying. "When you have a large ship on the rocks, and they tell you it's leaking oil, you know it is going to be bad, bad, bad." To deal with the unfolding crisis situation, Rawl, deciding not to waste time driving to his New York City office, began setting up conference calls from his home while his wife canceled Easter plans with the family.

Right from the start, Rawl says he "knew" that human error was to blame for the accident. Later, hearing that blood alcohol tests on the ship's captain, administered more than ten hours after the grounding, showed that the captain was legally drunk under Alaska law, Rawl said he was not surprised. As events that day unfolded, he began quickly to deal with the corporate-level issues related to the growing disaster. Three critical policy questions had to be answered: (1) What should Exxon's official stance be on the grounding? Should the company assume responsibility for the accident or what? (2) Should he, as chief executive of the company that employed the tanker's crew and owned the ship and the oil pouring into Prince William Sound, immediately go to Alaska to take charge of the situation and demonstrate Exxon's concern for what was happening? (3) How should information about the spill and subsequent containment and cleanup efforts be disseminated?

With regard to Exxon's official position on the grounding, the company's decision was to accept immediately full blame for what had happened as well as the responsibility for cleaning up the damage that was/would be done. As to the second question, Rawl's initial instinct was to go to Alaska. Later, however, he would be talked out of doing so by fellow Exxon executives. The rationale for not going was simple. If he went, he thought he would probably just be in the way and could serve the company's interests better from his office in New York. It was a decision that, in light of subsequent intense criticism, he would regret: "I wake up in the night questioning the decision to stay home."

His—Exxon's—decision to inform news organizations of events in Valdez on a "real time" basis (meaning that only Exxon employees in Valdez would provide information as it became available) also was a decision that he would come to regret. Reacting to charges that Exxon had manipulated and suppressed information back in the oil shortage days after the Arab embargo in the mid-1970s, Rawl said he wanted to get the information out: "At least you can't be accused of distorting data or slicking it up before it's presented to the press." But his new strategy still left the media frustrated and suspicious. Phone lines to Alaska were jammed constantly, Exxon officials there were often unavailable for comment, and the news conferences that took place in the "real time" off-hours made it next to impossible for the media networks and newspapers to present timely reports. "It just didn't work," Rawl says now.

Containment and Cleanup

From the beginning, Alyeska's attempts to contain and clean the oil slick from the waters and beaches of Prince William Sound were beset by many of the problems that often curse hastily put-together crisis organizations.

There was even some confusion about who was in charge: Eighteen hours after the spill, Exxon took over control from Alyeska.

Technical, Legal and Moral Issues

Alyeska's lack of preparedness and inability to cope with such a large spill almost immediately became the subjects of verbal sparring over technicalities and interpretations of the clean-up contingency plan. When the *Exxon Valdez* ran aground, the oil spill emergency barge was unloaded and in dry dock; it took twelve hours (the plan called for five) to mobilize and travel the 28 miles from the port in Valdez Harbor to the site of the accident. Further complicating things, barges and pumps which could have limited the spill by off-loading the remaining oil from the stricken ship were not available immediately. Because of these problems, Dennis Kelso, commissioner of the Alaska Department of Environmental Conservation, called Alyeska's emergency plan "the biggest piece of maritime fiction since *Moby Dick*." An Alyeska official responded to the charge: "This was a joint plan. We did exactly what the state [and federal governments] wanted. We did not deceive anyone, and we responded very well." Although Alyeska may have complied with the letter of the law (e.g., the joint plan never specified that the emergency barge had to be loaded), the plan, as everyone knew, was woefully inadequate for such an emergency.

As the spill spread, eventually oiling 1,200 miles of shoreline in the Sound to half-way out on the Alaska Peninsula (500 miles from the spill site), technological deficiencies and questions plagued decision makers. Fears of legal liability also seem to have played a major role in hindering early cleanup efforts. Lawyers representing Exxon, Alyeska, the state of Alaska, and the Coast Guard, for example, all urged their clients not to risk taking the initiative in cleanup efforts because of the potential for later liability claims. "The legal system crippled our ability to make decisions," Alaska's Governor Steve Cowper said at the time, "Protecting themselves [Exxon] from a lawsuit was more important than cleaning up oil." In response, Exxon President Raymond alleged that the state had deliberately delayed cleanup efforts so it could bolster its own legal case. "They have been preparing for litigation from day one," Raymond charged.

Soon after the accident, in an apparent move to shift blame for it, Exxon released to the press private information regarding Hazelwood's history of drinking problems, and then fired him. The reasons for the firing, however, were clarified later by Rawl: "A lot of the public and press think we fired him because we thought he was drunk on the ship, but we never said that, and we have cautioned people not to assume it. Hazelwood was terminated because he had violated company policies, such as not being on the bridge and for having consumed alcohol within four hours of boarding the ship." Predictably, the situation is viewed quite differently by Hazelwood who asserts that it is a commonly accepted practice for a ship's captain to issue simple instructions to the crew and then leave the bridge. When asked why Exxon and the state of Alaska both attempted to focus the blame for the incident on him, he replied that he did not know, but then said, "I could be a lightning rod, easy target, scapegoat to take the heat. I would say the same for the state of Alaska. They came after me, hammer and tongs, figuring I'd fold like a cheap suit. I imagine they're a bit surprised I didn't."

The outcome of all this sparring and legal wrangling was an expensive public relations war involving Exxon, the state of Alaska, and to some extent the former captain of the *Exxon Valdez*. However, more important perhaps than these was the withholding of important scientific data about the effects of the spill, collected by the many scientists on the scene, which could not be shared until later used in court.

Problems with Cleaning up the Oil

From the first day, Exxon argued that but for Alaska's bureaucratic fumbling it could have sprayed chemical dispersants (which reduce the surface tension of oil and allow it to break up into small droplets and scatter more easily into the water) on the spill that would have controlled the oil flow and subsequent damage. Not so, answers the state of Alaska, explaining that in the first few days after the spill when dispersants might have helped somewhat, Exxon had far too few chemicals available to do any good, and the calm seas would have prevented the chemicals from mixing throughly enough with the surrounding waters to be effective. There were also scientific questions raised about the toxicity of the dispersants and about their efficacy even under ideal conditions. The evidence shows that such chemically treated oil first scatters, then comes back together, sinks, resurfaces, and eventually washes ashore as tar balls; even though the oil seems to disappear, it does not go away.

Another severe problem for those trying to contain the spill was that the physical properties of an oil slick change over time. Although the most toxic parts of the oil evaporate in the first twenty hours or so, the remainder mixes with the salt water and sea debris so that after about fourteen days a heavy, thick, reddish-brown mousse is created. As the mousse collects even more debris, what does not amass on the beaches eventually can turn into an even thicker muck that will sink to the bottom. The thickening of the oil made it very difficult for the sixty skimmer vessels to vacuum the mess from the surface of the water and pump it into barges. According to Exxon's water cleanup coordinator Jim O'Brien, "There's an important thing people must realize in planning for a spill of this size: No amount of equipment will clean it all up, even if they give you a month's notice to get ready. Look at the expanse of water involved, and figure the time it takes to deploy boats and skimmers and support vessels at twelve knots. Skimmers need barges to collect their oil. Crews need food, ships need fuel, and somebody has to collect the garbage. And nothing works if the weather's bad."

The sticky mousse that ended up on the shores of Prince William Sound filled the nooks and crannies along the jagged coastal areas, saturating the surface and subsurfaces of the beaches, and pooling in some places to depths of over four feet. The strategy for cleaning these from the rocky beaches quickly focused on removing the gross oil and then letting the residue biodegrade over time. On the beaches of Prince William Sound where 90 percent of the oil went ashore, this meant that the mousse had to be scooped up, mopped, or blotted up before the rocks could be scrubbed semi-clean. Once this was done, the scrubbing often was done by hand but more generally by high pressure hoses. The hoses would shoot scalding water to loosen and then flush the oil, that had by now weathered to a substance somewhat like asphalt, back into the water where cold water hoses would direct it to off-shore skimmers. Another technique called bioremediation, used experimentally in places, involved spraying a special nitrogen-phosphorus fertilizer mix onto the shore in an attempt to stimulate oil-eating bacteria. It was hoped this would double the pace of nature's self-cleanup efforts.

This cleanup operation on the shorelines of Prince William Sound was not, however, without its share of controversies. Each technique used to clean the beaches had critics. For example, some believed that because it tended to kill the fish and surviving micro-organisms, the scalding water used to scrub the beaches created worse ecological problems than the oil. Critics also complained that bioremediation, although it seemed to work in the few areas where it was tried, would leave unsightly, non-toxic asphalt hydrocarbons to stain the beaches, and would cause an undesirable growth in the Sound's plankton population. There were complaints that the debris and garbage created by the cleanup crews were in themselves ecological disasters. There were serious complaints also that the workers sent to Alaska were poorly trained and that the conditions in which those workers toiled were hazardous to their health—they virtually lived in oil-soaked clothing for long periods, constantly had oil on their faces and hands, and were often not provided with breathing protectors. It is well known that exposure to oil and its vapors can lead to nausea, breathing difficulties, rashes, kidney and nervous system damage, as well as cancer.

Perhaps the major criticism of cleanup efforts, however, is that they serve no other purpose than the public relations interests of the principals (Exxon, the state of Alaska, and the Coast Guard) responsible for the mess in the first place. Many believe that, beyond the initial wildlife kills and the temporary (an estimated three to six years) destruction of the scenery, the lasting effects of the spill on the environment will be minimal. The cleanup had little beneficial effect on the environment, possibly added to the adverse consequences and, as a practical matter, amounted to nothing more than a (multi)billion dollar public relations campaign to assuage the anger of the people of Alaska, environmentalists, the larger general public, and Congress. The oil industry, in particular, had a lot at stake in public opinion. They greatly feared the potential political damage any adverse publicity would have on requests for further off-shore drilling rights and for permission to explore for gas and oil in other environmentally sensitive areas in Alaska and elsewhere in the United States. One of the great ironies of the cleanup effort is perhaps best expressed on the most popular t-shirt in Valdez during the summer of 1989: "Cleanup '89. It's not just a job, it's a ——ing waste of time."

Exxon paid out anywhere from $1 to $3 billion (there have been several different numbers reported), while employing approximately 11,500 people in the cleanup effort. In addition, Exxon compensated Alaskan fishermen some $200,000 for lost income due to the spill. Who can estimate the value of 980 otters, 138 eagles and 33,126 other birds killed?

As the cleanup operation shut down on September 15, 1989, in advance of the harsh Alaskan winter, Exxon loudly recited its list of accomplishments: 60,000 barrels of recovered oil and 1,087 miles of oiled beach now environmentally stable. The state of Alaska countered by reporting that the cleanup actually had recovered fewer than 30,000 barrels of oil and that only about 118 miles of beaches were safe for wildlife and new vegetation. Despite their release of an ambiguously worded memo (on July 19, 1989) that seemed to state that, the job being finished, the company would not return in the spring to resume cleanup efforts—a memo that generated enormous public outrage—Exxon returned to Prince William Sound on May 1, 1990, to do what was necessary, as established by Coast Guard recommendations, to make things right.

Sources

Associated Press report, "Conoco Alters Stand on Tankers," *South Bend Tribune,* April 11, 1990.

Behar, R., "Exxon Strikes Back: Interview with Lawrence Rawl," *Time,* March 26, 1990, pp. 62-63.

Byrne, J. A., "The Rebel Shaking up Exxon," *Business Week,* July 18, 1988, pp. 104-111.

DiIanni, D., "The Big Spill," for *NOVA;* PBS air-date: February 27, 1990; 1990 WGBH Educational Foundation; transcript by Journal Graphics, 267 Broadway, New York, NY 10007.

Hodgson, B., "Alaska's Big Spill: Can the Wilderness Heal?" *National Geographic,* January 1990, pp. 2-43.

Interview with Joseph Hazelwood conducted by Connie Chung, telecast on *Saturday Night with Connie Chung,* March 31, 1990.

Satchell, M., and Carpenter, B., "A Disaster That Wasn't," *U.S. News & World Report,* September 18, 1989, pp. 60-69.

Solomon, J., "Strategies for Handling the Arrest of an Employee," *Wall Street Journal,* March 29, 1990.

Stigler, G., "What an Oil Spill Is Worth," *Wall Street Journal,* April 17, 1990.

Sullivan, A., "Exxon's Restructuring in the Past Is Blamed for Recent Accidents: Cost cuts in '86 helped profit, but did they make spills, refinery fire more likely?" *Wall Street Journal,* March 16, 1990.

Sullivan, A., "Rawl Wishes He'd Visited Valdez Sooner: Exxon Chief Regrets Actions Right after Oil Spill," *Wall Street Journal,* June 6, 1989.

Tobias, M., "Black Tide," for the *Discovery Channel;* air-date: March 18, 1990.

Tuttle, J., "Anatomy of an Oil Spill," for *FRONTLINE;* PBS air-date: March 20, 1990; 1990 WGBH Educational Foundation; transcript by Journal Graphics, 267 Broadway, New York, NY 10007.

Wall Street Journal, "Oil Spill Cleanups Still Protect Workers Poorly, Unions Say," April 10, 1990.

Wall Street Journal, "Review and Outlook: Cleaning Up Oil," March 30, 1990.

Suggested Readings

Douglas, M., and Wildavsky, A., *Risk and Culture: An Essay on the Selection of Technological and Environmental Dangers* (Berkeley, CA: University of California Press, 1982). Important reading because of its provocative insights on the role of cultural factors in perception, risk assessment, and strategy decisions.

Frost, P.J., Mitchell, V.F., and Nord, W.R., *Managerial Reality: Balancing Technique, Practice, and Values.* Glenview, IL: Scott, Foresman/Little, Brown Higher Education (1990). An insightful set of readings which focus on discrepancies between what is taught about management and what is experienced by managers in the so-called "real world."

Goodpaster, K.E., and Sayre, K.M., eds., *Ethics and Problems of the 21st Century* (Notre Dame: University of Notre Dame Press, 1979). Leading moral philosophers examine environmental and social issues.

Jackall, R., *Moral Mazes: The World of Corporate Managers* (New York: Oxford University Press, 1988). A compelling account of managerial life and the foundations of ethics/moral behavior in modern organizations.

Passmore, J., *Man's Responsibility for Nature* (New York: Charles Scribner's Sons, 1974). A classic in environmental ethics, which discusses the kind of moral and metaphysical response needed to resolve the ecological crisis.

Singer, P., *Animal Liberation* (New York: New York Review, 1975). A highly influential utilitarian defense of animal rights.

Weick, K.E., *The Social Psychology of Organizing* (Reading, MA: Addison-Wesley, 1979). Karl Weick's classic book exploring how we make sense of, learn from, and act on the things we individually and/or collectively decide are the realities of organizational life.

Seven

Stories and Culture in Business Life

John W. Houck

In a seminar recently, I asked a young man to give his judgments about the American Business System. He is a business administration senior, bright and hard-working, idealistic and responsible. In the vernacular of a few years ago, he is a "straight" type. Yet he betrayed his demeanor by commencing a stream-of-consciousness recitation, slowly and firmly:

> Maybe I fear going out into the system, but I see it as being too large, very impersonal, too deaf to the needs of the individual. Everything is judged by its contribution to profit. Business PR is a smokescreen; look at equal opportunity and the ecology—how late business was on those. Business manipulates the consumer and the regulators. Government and business are too frequently in collusion, or asleep. Why, [and here he searched for the right term for his purpose, either to suggest hypocrisy or good intentions turned sour in practice] it is like a Dr. Jekyll and Mr. Hyde!

It is not good that a young person is so pessimistic. For he sees business, his intended field, in violation of Alfred North Whitehead's dictum that a great society is one in which its men and women of business think greatly of their role. He sees himself "condemned" to a career with an extremely low ethical horizon. It is not enough to offer consolation. Our task is to provide for this young person realistic hope that he can live out humane and religious values in business life. Our possible answer to him is the subject of this discussion.

The Theme of Two Cities

To the question, What is it that the humanities can say to such a person? The consensual answer is, "Very little!" This is surprising as the humanities, including religious thought, claim to speak to the theme of an overarching world view about life and possible strategies about how we should live. But the humanities, in military parlance, appear to have yielded the highways and cities, thereby being reduced to studied aloofness or to a sharply adversarial stance. Meanwhile, the business and technocratic mentality picks away at targets of opportunity such as computers, telecommunications and biogenetics. They are fashioning new civilizations which, with irresistible momentum, determine our future and lives. Peter Drucker reminds us: "You in business don't market a product; you market a civilization."

There is a substantial literature which argues that a deep chasm separates the business mentality and its critics. We are told:

> No man can serve two masters: for either he will hate the one, and love the other; or else he will hold to the one, and despise the other. (Matthew 6:24)

The biblical writer Matthew is quite *certain* about our inability to serve both God and mammon. Later, St. Augustine likewise will see irreconcilable conflicts growing out of what we deign to love. There is a worldly city, Babylon, which "flowered from a selfish love" and is marked by excessive interest in "belongings" of this world. The other city, Jerusalem, was founded on the love of God and is marked by profound "longings" by its inhabitants for God. There appears to be precious little middle ground in the Augustinian view between the two possible objects of our love, God or self, *caritas* or *cupidatas*.

In his classic study, *The Protestant Ethic and the Spirit of Capitalism*, Max Weber carefully traced the role of a powerful religious tradition, Calvinism and its offshoots—including puritanism—in the birth of capitalism. And although this tracing is the stuff of history's "how we moderns arrived at our present situation," there is an important obser-vation of Weber's:

> ...the intensity of the search for the Kingdom of God commenced gradually to pass over into sober economic virtue; the religious roots died out slowly, giving way to utilitarian worldliness.

In the 1950s, Allen Ginsberg, a leader of the Beat Generation, published his famous *Howl.* Ginsberg saw us dominated by business

values. He characterized U.S. culture by giving it the name of the hated
deity Moloch:

> Moloch whose mind is pure machinery! Moloch whose blood is
> running money! Moloch whose fingers are ten armies! Moloch whose
> breast is a cannibal dynamo! Moloch whose ear is a smoking tomb![1]

Norman Mailer, in his *Armies of the Night*,[2] saw the religious person
working in corporate America caught in a vise which would split the mind
from the soul. For Mailer, the heart of the humanities and religious
thought is mystery, but at the center of business technology is a
detestation of mystery. And mystery, in the words of William
Wordsworth, requires hearing "the still, sad music of humanity" which
is not "harsh or grating" but still has "ample power to chasten and
subdue."

Today, business corporations are becoming huge knowledge facto-
ries of specialists, pursuing bits of information and technical competen-
cies. This is portrayed effectively in Tracy Kidder's volume, *The Soul of
a New Machine*,[3] in which a team of specialists raced to beat out rival
companies, and the Japanese, in the design of an advanced new computer.
In a sense, the whole process is reduced to a sporting event! The team
won the contest but would soon be reconstituted with different specialists
to start out again: "It was just another routine day down at debugging
headquarters." What is eerie about all this is the silence on the cultural
or ethical goodness or badness of the new machine. "We needed it to fill
out the product line." The knowledge factory rarely intrudes questions
of the humane life or fidelity to the Kingdom of God as it pursues the
rich material life through technical competence.

Historically, Judeo-Christian religions—evoking a common tradition—have had a vision of what constitutes the good life: love of God
and service to others, as well as the attitudes, or virtues, that should flow
from the vision. The Judeo-Christian would go further and claim that
his or her religious view of the good life is deeper, more satisfying, and
more "true" than any claimant. Does all this lead up to a fundamental
impasse? Some observers have suggested as much:

> The personality profile of successful businesspeople...is not calculated
> to warm the heart of moralists or teachers of spiritual perfection....Many
> theologians claim God is not to be found in the marketplace among
> the rich and powerful but at the edge, with the poor and the powerless.

Being committed to monetary values in order to succeed in business places (a corporate executive) in a psychological stance which pulls (him or her) sharply and powerfully away from the exigencies of Christianity. One simply cannot serve two different masters—God and mammon.[4]

I am sure there were trustworthy, reliable, faithful persons who acknowledged their implicit obligations to communities, customers, and others, and who acted in a praiseworthy way in this regard. But such a person within a corporate structure surely has often had to subsume his or her personal morality to the requirements of the "office."[5]

A few years ago Peter Cohen wrote a book, *The Gospel According to the Harvard Business School*,[6] which detailed the perspective of the new managerial elite in our corporations. He was deadly serious in his use of the word "Gospel," for what he described was the formation of a large cadre of young men and women who have a sense of reality nurtured in this Gospel, which is in contrast to other world views such as the religious, humanistic, romantic or scientific. This world view, although relatively young as intellectual or faith traditions go, stems from the cultural ideas (and tangible success) of the last two hundred years of the Industrial Revolution. The humanities, therefore, are seen in the utilitarian role of "helping us to communicate better" or "clearing up this writing problem" but certainly not helping us to answer the two questions: "What's it all about?" or "How should we live?"

"It Takes a Helluva Lot of Competence to Do Good!"

Let me tell a story to illustrate how the humanities and religious thought might impact on the career and ambitions of a typical middle manager. I like stories because they are our earliest manifestations of wanting to know and to understand: "Daddy, or Mommy, tell me a story." Also, unlike a theory which can let you know the world without changing it, a story helps you with the world by changing it through changing yourself.

• • • • •

James Mitchell was in a quandary. He needed a new building for the hand and power tool plant he ran—the Miller Falls Company of Greenfield, Massachusetts. His first tendency was to move to the Sunbelt and take advantage of increased space, lower taxes and reduced wage rates. On the other hand, such a move would leave 700 people without jobs in this small New England town.

At that time, the northeastern states had suffered such economic blows too often in recent years. They were beginning to fight back. As Jim Mitchell started his reluctant search for a site in North Carolina, state and local officials near the plant got wind of the situation. Leaders in the business community formed an economic development corporation to acquire and finance new property. Mitchell listened to their plans, and cautioned them about how difficult it was to meet the competition.

Dealing with Ingersoll-Rand, the parent company, and with the union, became his next tasks. A suitable site and wage rates closer to those in the south were both a must before the board of directors would consider approval of the proposal.

Mitchell turned to the union and asked for a wage reduction and for changes in the plant's wage incentive program. These requests were met with a flat rejection.

His next move was to take his cause directly to the workers. He walked out on the plant floor—a place now charged with fear and emotion. Jim stopped operations and called everyone together. He told them that unless the union agreed to talk, they would all be losers.

Shortly thereafter, the union agreed to bargain and, after three arduous months, they approved a four-year contract which Mitchell took to the Ingersoll-Rand board. It was accepted pending location of a site at the right cost.

The place was located finally in Deerfield, Massachusetts, a small neighboring community. With the unflagging determination of some local bankers, financing was arranged and the purchase was started very closely by the start of construction.

Was the company just bluffing about leaving? Some of the union members thought so, but Jim Mitchell insisted he did what he had to do to keep the plant in Massachusetts. He says, "It wasn't a bluff. It wasn't intended to be blackmail. It was a business decision." But beneath the calm demeanor here was a manager who took a long and difficult path to save a plant and maybe a community.[7]

•   •   •   •   •

What are we to say about this narrative? Certainly, as I have recounted it to a number of successful managers across the country, I have been met with looks of amazement. "It is unusual for a company to reverse its decision to relocate a plant." "I count on one hand the number of times this might have happened in a background of hundreds of plant moves." From my anti-business friends, equally incredulous reactions: "What do you expect from *those* people!" They assume this is a statistical fluke. Even Attila the Hun had his moments. But the point is not whether it happens many or few times, but what we can learn about life in corporate America, and about how we should live.

Corporations have an image and a value system all their own, which impacts heavily on men and women in the managerial ranks. The corporate images and values dictate what constitutes a good performance or a bad one, a successful or unsuccessful career. Certainly, one way to gain insight into business is to ask about the images and values that seem to be guiding life in the corporate world: *What Makes the Manager Run?*

Frankly, business has never recovered from Budd Schulberg's nearly fifty-year-old novel, *What Makes Sammy Run?*,[8] a bitterly satirical book about the ambitious Sammy who cuts friends and steps on the weak as he reaches for the next rung on the ladder. For too many who reject business out of hand, the caricature, Sammy, is forever their window to understanding the business world and its people: "Ambition and money are everything, and the cost in ethics, loyalty, good taste be damned!" And although we all know a few *Sammies*, they are as far from the norm in business today as sexual cads are the norm in academe. More importantly, there is a hopelessness about Sammy. He is so distasteful that no one would waste his or her time talking ethics with *that* kind of person.

An Ethical Corporate Culture Is Critical

It would be helpful to consider the contrast of what Jim Mitchell did in the *Wall Street Journal* article and another story which could have been written. Supposing Jim Mitchell were part of an organization that prided itself on performance, effectiveness, growth, result. This organization put great pressure on its people to perform and to excel; further, they were encouraged to see themselves in competition with others. In less than subtle ways, people were paired up in career heats to ascertain which one could handle it. We might imagine Jim Mitchell responding in the manner of the image of a King of the Mountain, the popular children's game where the goal is to get to the top of a hill and remain there, pushing off all competitors. Only here, no physical force is used, but performance, toughness and self-discipline are the logic of the game.

The image, King of the Mountain, fits well with the Success Ethic which holds sway among much of America's elite. The values held by people in the upper levels of middle management are the results of a long orientation and formation, going back to high school, if not grade school, preaching the virtues of hard work and achievement which lead to happiness, power, status, security and money. Success is never guaranteed, however, as this comes through competition with peers in climbing the corporate ladder. *Upward mobility by testing and achievement is the key to success in the multi-layered modern corporation.*

In an important article on Corporate Culture, *Business Week* described one company which prides itself on encouraging competitive types. "To keep everyone on their toes, a 'creative tension' is continually nurtured among departments...The staff is kept lean and managers are moved to new jobs constantly, which results in people working long hours and engaging in political maneuvering...." The article points out that in such a culture, less competitive managers, or managers from a different mold are deliberately weeded out.

James Mitchell could have followed the dictates of this corporate culture by reasoning: It will be an important accomplishment on my résumé, overseeing the building and staffing of a completely new facility. As *Business Week* put it:

> Just as tribal cultures have totems and taboos that dictate how each member will act toward fellow members and outsiders, so does a corporation's culture influence employees' actions toward customers, competitors, suppliers, and one another. Sometimes the rules are written out. More often they are tacit. Most often, they are laid down by a strong founder and hardened by success into custom.[9]

Of course, any executive worth his or her salt would appreciate what this move would mean to the medium-sized New England town, a loss of seven hundred jobs and a ripple effect loss of $35 million in economic activity. But Jim could quiet his conscience by thinking: "The opportunities for me are great, and anyway this isn't the first plant to ever relocate, and it won't be the last!"

The Servant Image

But James Mitchell did not follow the logic of the imagery of a King of the Mountain. Although there is no way of knowing what he was actually thinking, it is helpful to use what he did as subject for ethical reflection. I would argue that to live a full and ethical life means that some of the important humane and religious images are used to interpret experience and guide our lives in the business world. For instance, we might ask ourselves about the values and virtues we could uncover from the struggles of Virgil's hero, Aeneas, to persevere and to build a great city, Rome. While we struggle today to build great corporate organizations, we can learn from Aeneas. He is the earliest of our cultural heroes to represent *the civic virtues of duty, courage in decision making and the need for a strong community.*

We might also ask ourselves about the meaning of Machiavelli's *Prince.* Machiavelli wanted his leader (or in today's terms—manager) to bring a hardheaded realism to the decision making about building a society where human beings could grow strong, wise and productive— in spite of themselves. Both Aeneas and the Prince point to the value of service to others as at least a partial answer to the question: How should we live?

In the religious tradition, we find a similar response. For instance, supposing our manager was using an image in his life which was consciously biblical. Could it set the context for his deliberations about the plant closing? He might see himself, based on religious conviction, as a Servant, which would mean he sees himself as a person *and* a manager, *thrust into the hopes and ambitions of the world, and yet having a calling to realize God's love and justice.* The Jesus Story,[10] here interpreted as a model of one who came to serve and *not* to be served, can affect and even change our manager's perception of self and personal ambition. It can also change the business world about him.

Our manager, because of his appropriation of the Servant Image, wants to save the jobs in the New England town. Therefore, he can be described as a person of good will, but he must have the co-requisite competence to save the jobs. Competence in this case means: (1) preparing financial analysis for the corporate directors to demonstrate that a new plant in New England would be competitive in performance with one in the Sunbelt; (2) convincing town and state officials to take action (land acquisition, building bonds, etc.) comparable to the Sunbelt's proven record in luring and welcoming industry; and (3) finally, to convince workers and their union leaders to accept wage restraints to bring labor costs in line with Sunbelt rates. As one senior executive observed, "In today's complexity, it takes a helluva lot of competence to do good, and business people are frequently the ones best able to get the job done." It would not be surprising if at bleak moments Jim Mitchell did not admit to himself: "Is it all worth it? Why not chuck it all and go South?" But he did not and a new plant was built, saving the jobs and keeping that area from sliding further into regional depression.

Stories, like that of Jim Mitchell's, can suggest the images and values from both the humane and religious traditions which can challenge the logic of our ordinary business ways, both on the level of our personal response to "how should we live" and on the level of social and institutional structures and values. But to challenge does not mean necessarily to reject; it does point to the possibilities for creative, critical action by managers despite the limitations of "reality." It does point to greater openness in business thinking and values. Yet, none of this suggests a rejection of managerial competence and effectiveness. Ethical managers will just have to learn to do both, that is, be ethical and be competent.

Notes

1. Allen Ginsberg, "Howl," *Howl, and Other Poems* (San Francisco: City Lights Pocket Bookshop, 1956), ii. 5-6.

2. Norman Mailer, *The Armies of the Night: History as a Novel and the Novel as History* (New York: New American Library, 1968), *passim*, p. 188.

3. Tracey Kidder, *The Soul of a New Machine* (Boston: Little, Brown and Company, 1981).

4. Denis A. Goulet, "Goals in Conflict," *The Judeo-Christian Vision and the Modern Corporation*, eds. Oliver F. Williams and John W. Houck (Notre Dame, IN: University of Notre Dame Press, 1982), pp. 221-225.

5. James M. Gustafson and Elmer W. Johnson, "The Corporate Leader and the Ethical Resources of Religion: A Dialogue," *The Judeo-Christian Vision*, pp. 309-311.

6. Peter Cohen, *The Gospel According to the Harvard Business School: The Education of America's Managerial Elite* (New York: Doubleday and Company, 1973).

7.   Liz Roman Gallese, "Bucking the Trend: A New England Town Stops a Big Employer from Moving to South," *Wall Street Journal*, January 9, 1978, p. 1.

8. Budd Schulberg, *What Makes Sammy Run?* (New York: Penguin Books, 1978).

9.   "Corporate Culture: The Hard-to-Change Values that Spell Success or Failure," *Business Week* (New York), October 27, 1980, p. 148.

10.   Oliver F. Williams and John W. Houck, *Full Value: Cases in Christian Business Ethics* (San Francisco: Harper and Row, 1978), p. 55.

Eight

The Business of Storytelling and Storytelling in Business

Dennis P. McCann

The rediscovery of the role of narrative in interpreting religious and moral experience is clearly one of the most significant changes of the past decade in the way American theologians approach the field of religious ethics. As in most important breakthroughs, in hindsight this process seems to involve recovering the forgotten obvious. How could we have overlooked it? Yet overlook it many did until a happy combination of relatively arcane methodological studies in hermeneutics, and grassroots manifestoes demanding recognition of the distinctive religious and moral experience of a whole range of oppressed and minority communities made it clear that, whatever their aspirations toward systematic understanding, theologians risk betraying the religious traditions and communities to which they have pledged their loyalties if they continue to neglect the narrative bases of their commitments.

Yet the recovery of the significance of narrative in theology might not have made much of an impact on our understanding of religious ethics were it not for the provocative interventions of philosopher Alasdair MacIntyre and theologian Stanley Hauerwas.[1] MacIntyre's *After Virtue*[2] not only demonstrated the futility of doing ethics on the basis of the so-called "standard account of morality," but also outlined an agenda for understanding ethics as the cultivation of virtue within communities of memory still oriented to visions of the good life. The practice of virtue called for by MacIntyre emphasized the importance of the communities' narrative traditions. Hauerwas's major statement, *The Peaceable Kingdom*,[3] showed how biblical narratives help us not only to envision the world in distinctively Christian imagery but also to understand the ways in which the religious truth-claims raised by these traditions can and must shape the basic orientation of Christian ethics.

Though not every theologian is prepared to accept the strong animus against liberal modernity that MacIntyre and Hauerwas seem to share, their efforts clearly have shifted the assumptions governing the discussion of ethics in the United States today. Any account of morality that neglects the significance of narrative now commonly is regarded as seriously defective.

Unfortunately, the field of business ethics, as represented by philosophers like Richard DeGeorge, Manuel Velasquez, Tom Beauchamp and Norman Bowie, has continued to develop either in ignorance of the newer narrative approaches or, more likely, in the mistaken belief that such approaches are only marginally relevant for understanding morality in business. Indeed, the textbooks authored by these philosophers are among the clearest examples still to be found of the paradigm rejected by MacIntyre, Hauerwas and others. There is, of course, one impressive departure from the standard account of morality in the field of business ethics, the pioneering work of Oliver Williams and John Houck, first outlined in *Full Value: Cases in Christian Business Ethics.*[4] Rather than once more rake over the old chestnuts about the inadequacies of the philosophers just mentioned,[5] I want to take this opportunity to interpret the not yet fully realized promise of *Full Value.* In this paper I will attempt to develop the leads indicated by Willliams and Houck in the following manner:

(1) I will offer an interpretation of *Full Value* that is both appreciative and critical: appreciative of its ground-breaking attempt to demonstrate the relevance of Christian narrative for orienting the personal character of businesspeople, and critical of two key limitations. The first limitation is its adoption of a narrowly evangelical approach to the Christian story and, the second, its apparent failure to move beyond personal character formation to the constitutive role of narrative in the formation of corporate cultures in business. Unless this social dimension of storytelling in business is understood fully, and unless Christianity's substantive impact upon business values is conceived through stories that are more responsive to the ironies and moral ambiguities of institutional development, the role of narrative in Christian business ethics will remain needlessly restricted.

(2) I will try to follow the actual example of Williams and Houck's case studies by offering a theological interpretation of a series of contemporary business narratives. Michael Maccoby's *The Gamesman,*[6] with some modification, provided the framework within which *Full*

Value approached the business stories selected for scrutiny. The question is whether Maccoby's study still captures the range of characters defining the business ethos today, in the wake of the "Roaring Eighties." I have chosen four books to represent today's business stories—marked, as they are, by the rebirth of entrepreneurialism and the relatively brief cultural ascendancy of the financial markets and their recent chilling contractions. Two of the books are personal autobiographies and two are journalistic studies of newly emerging groups of businesspeople, and all of them published recently: Michael Lewis's *Liar's Poker*,[7] John H. Johnson's *Succeeding Against the Odds*,[8] Michael Meyer's *The Alexander Complex*[9] and Anne B. Fisher's *Wall Street Women*.[10]

Based on a survey of these books, I will argue that businesspeople do not need to be sold on a narrative approach to understanding morality, for storytelling is clearly the preferred way by which individuals are socialized into the ethos of business as a whole as well as into particular corporate cultures. What is called for, therefore, is not another apology for narrative but a critical evaluation of the stories already communicated in the world of business. I will try to illustrate the possibilities for such an evaluation by using story patterns taken from the whole of Christian tradition to sketch a deliberately hopeful experiment in interpretation. I hope to suggest that beyond any theologically forced choice between religious and secular values lies the central theme of the Augustinian perspective in Catholic tradition, namely, the vision of a Divine Comedy in which grace builds upon nature, often in ironic and subtle ways. If this story line is still capable of communicating an authentically Christian vision of the world in which we work out our salvation, it must be as capable of being discerned in the stories of businesspeople and institutions as it is in any other walk of life.

How to Get Full Value from Full Value

Full Value: Cases in Christian Business Ethics is a deceptively simple book. It modestly presents a number of radical theses about the nature of the Christian life and how it might be lived in business. For Williams and Houck rightly contend that, in principle at least, there is no discontinuity between the kind of moral reasoning done by businesspeople and that sustained in religious communities. If storytelling has an important role to play both in communicating basic orientations ("vision") and in shaping character in the one, then, surely, storytelling will play a similar role in the other. A program in Christian business ethics, thus, is not simply an attempt to explicate the meaning of biblical stories for businesspeople but, more precisely, to use the leads given in these stories to help people create or interpret their own stories in business.

To facilitate this convergence of storytelling perspectives, Williams and Houck offer a set of seven doctrinal abstractions or "values" they believe convey the distinctive characteristics of the Christian way of life. These abstractions—"power over individuals as service," "power over nature as stewardship," "wealth and property as an opportunity for increased service... [and]...a possible obstacle to salvation," "happiness as achieved by following God's intentions," "justice as the right of each person to the means of leading a human life," "deferred gratification," and "time as reverence for God"—explicitly derive their meaning from familiar biblical stories told and retold in the Christian communities. By rendering these narrative perspectives as abstractions, Williams and Houck, like all theologians, are seeking to extend the claims implicit in Christian storytelling to the wider world beyond the direct influence of the communities of faith. Once regarded as a particular set of "values," these perspectives can be compared with other sets available in society at large. Williams and Houck thus clearly hope to stimulate a confrontation in which Christians committed to the perspectives opened up in the biblical stories come to experience their lives as a "struggle to bring the values of the Kingdom of God into this world."[11] The point is neither to abandon the world to those who live by other values, nor to embrace it presumptuously, but to reinforce the believer's hope of embodying in his or her own life a creative tension uniting the one with the other.

The terms of that struggle are given already in the general contrasts by which Williams and Houck clarify the meaning of the set of seven "Judeo-Christian values."[12] The seven "contrasting values"—"power over individuals as domination and control," power over nature as a "mandate to produce a maximum of consumer goods," "wealth and property as the measure of a person's worth," "happiness as achieved through acquiring possessions," "justice as the protection of property already possessed," "immediate gratification," and "time as money"—are not timelessly universal in their portrayal of unredeemed worldliness, but are a specific indictment of the most frequently deplored excesses of a modern capitalistic society. At times, Williams and Houck seem to be making the wholly debatable assumption that the world of business, in fact, is characterized by this set of values. At other times, the situation is admitted to be "highly complex."[13] Nevertheless, this set is used to picture the general features of the context in which the Christian's daily struggle continues.

For more specific descriptions of the world of business, Williams and Houck expand upon the four character types discerned by Michael Maccoby in his study of business executives and the stories they tell about themselves.[14] Maccoby's four types are: "(1) The Jungle Fighter, one who will do most anything to look good; (2) The Craftsman, one who takes pride in the work; (3) The Gamesman, one who thrives on a fast-paced, competitive game; and (4) The Company Man, one who is concerned about the long-range values of the institution."[15] Williams and Houck's list of six "Master Images in the Business World" omits Maccoby's "Jungle Fighter," and adds "The Millionaire," one whose business activity is dedicated to the pursuit of financial success; "The Captain on the Bridge," one whose business activity is geared to appeasing the variety of competing interest groups by which he sees himself besieged; and "The King of the Mountain," who, much like "The Jungle Fighter," thrives on exercising power over others.[16] Since, as Williams and Houck insist, none of these is necessarily "incompatible with a master image from the Bible,"[17] the struggle between the Judeo-Christian and the contrasting set of values goes on, or can go on, in each of them.

Nevertheless, it is clear that the "Master Images from the Bible" are more likely to take root and transform some of these six more readily than others. My impression from using *Full Value* in the classroom for at least five years is that the hardly exhaustive list of Christian images sketched by Williams and Houck—"A Pilgrim of the People of God," "An Heir to the Kingdom of God," and "Servant of the Lord"—have more affinities with "The Craftsperson," "The Company Person" and "The Captain on the Bridge" than with "The Millionaire," "The King of the Mountain," and "The Gamesman." The latter have in common narrowly competitive or crudely individualistic descriptions of business success, while the former seem to embody broader social visions not only of success but also of the very purpose of business. I remember being quite depressed by this discovery for it suggested that a Christian approach to business ethics, despite Williams and Houck's assurances to the contrary, was possible only within a limited range of character types, perhaps among those regarded at that time as least likely to achieve significant success in business.

This first disappointment led to further discoveries that helped me pinpoint precisely where my own perspective differed from that of Williams and Houck. As I understand these differences, they do not call into question Williams and Houck's pioneering insights into the role of narrative-based images in character formation or the ways in which Christian imagery can be used as leads for evaluating, challenging and, perhaps, transforming the stories businesspeople tell about themselves. Our differences are substantive rather than methodological, at least at first. They revolve around the adequacy of Williams and Houck's characterization of the contrast between the values embedded in the biblical stories and those represented by the world. Beyond this, they involve the institutional dimension of both sets of values and how an adequate understanding of this dimension may serve to soften, or even overcome entirely, the stipulated contrast. One way of focusing these concerns is to ask whether, strictly for business reasons, a corporation typically has any stake in which of the six "Master Images" may come to dominate the imaginations of its managers. If the objectives of a business corporation are more likely to be met by managers displaying affinities with "The Craftsperson," "The Company Person," and "The Captain on the Bridge" than with the other subset of crudely individualistic types, then the relationship between the Christian way of life and working for a business corporation may not be as confrontational as Williams and Houck seem to depict it.

Let me explain, first, my theological reservations about Williams and Houck's contrast between the two sets of values: the allegedly Judeo-Christian one and that of an unredeemed world. By trying to demonstrate the distinctive characteristics of the Christian vision of the world, they have fallen into the trap of ignoring all but a narrow range of biblical texts, primarily the New Testament parables of the Kingdom of God. True enough, such narratives do give us the essential teachings of Jesus of Nazareth, to the extent these are available. But by taking them out of their historical context to emphasize the religious and moral challenge they represent, Williams and Houck ignore the fact that these stories are inherently and deliberately disorienting, that they invite their hearers and readers to break with convention and institutional routine and to embark upon a new adventure whose ultimate institutional contours are only vaguely discerned in the imagery of the Kingdom.

Williams and Houck's range of biblical stories, in short, represents only one segment in the process of forming either Christian communities or moral character within them. The missing segments, of course, are the histories of both Israel and the church, by no means just the Roman Catholic church but the traditions of all branches of Christianity, as well as Judaism, that have tried to bear witness to the Kingdom of God while living faithfully in this world. What an awareness of these extended narrative contexts might supply is models for actually living out the creative tension to which the New Testament parables mostly just invite us. What range of images of institutional and social responsibility is disclosed by the extended traditions of the biblical communities of faith? How is power to be exercised, and wealth to be managed, by persons who must not only strive for faithfulness to the Kingdom of God but also exercise leadership in a world that only partially manifests this vision?

I suggest that such questions of responsibility will force us to consider a broader range of biblical and post-biblical narratives than those emphasized by Williams and Houck. One who would exercise leadership in business might do well to consider in detail the stories of Abraham, Moses, Joshua and David, or Judith and Ruth, with these questions in mind. In the New Testament there are the stories of Peter and Paul in the Acts of the Apostles and in various Epistles. They testify as to the struggle to create a religious community independent of traditional Judaism yet capable of enduring beyond the deaths of their founders who followed Jesus during his brief ministry. Beyond these biblical narratives, but in stories that are often patterned by them, there are the resources of tradition, for example, "The Lives of the Saints," especially those of St. Augustine of Hippo, St. Benedict of Nursia, St. Catherine of Siena, St. Theresa of Avila and, more recently, St. Vincent de Paul and St. Louise de Marillac. These saints were either the innovative founders of great religious enterprises or institutional reformers who saw their mission as the renewal rather than the abandonment of our common life.

Among the ways in which one's Christian vision will be enriched by working with these narratives is a more realistic sense of how to accommodate the vision to the constraints of worldly responsibility. Here one will find mentors in the indispensable art of compromise, subtle guides on when to stand firm and when to yield to the ways of the world. There will be lessons also in patience, prudence and perseverance, qualities of leadership that often seem to be eclipsed by the urgency of the Kingdom proclamations. Above all, one will find a realization that the Christian communities' situation in the world already has been shaped decisively by Western civilization's responses to the events proclaimed in the New Testament and that what we regard as the world is no longer simply unredeemed but partially transformed by the witness of preceding generations of believers. In short, one will find a more profound sense of the mystery of the Incarnation than could possibly have been expressed in the New Testament itself.

The history of the church is particularly instructive about the difficulties that any Christian leader can expect to encounter in trying to remain faithful to the Founder's vision while responding to the constraints imposed by the normal patterns of organizational behavior. If, as Peter Drucker once observed, the task of management is to help ordinary people do extraordinary things, the challenge is no less difficult in churches than in business corporations. Indeed, a detailed understanding of the vicissitudes of church history might provide Christian business people not only with a deeper appreciation of the challenges of sound management, but also with the consolation that stems from realizing that failure to live up to the vision is just as common in religious communities as it is in business. Such insights do not render invalid the abstract contrast that Williams and Houck draw between Judeo-Christian values and the alternative set representing an unredeemed world. But as the institutional leadership of both ancient Israel and the church came to realize, often to their bitter regret, they do suggest that the struggle is one that goes on within the communities of faith and not just one that is brought from outside by these communities into an unredeemed world.

From a theological perspective focused upon the Incarnation, business corporations may be regarded as already implicated in the history of Christian redemption, and just as ambiguously as have all the churches.[18] If business is thus no more worldly than the churches already have proven themselves to be, then the struggle to live by the vision of the Kingdom of God can and must proceed in both institutional locations with an equally profound sense of irony and humility. Therefore, despite the impression created by Williams and Houck's apparently evangelical bias, I must affirm that the church has as much to learn from the world as vice-versa. A Christian approach to business ethics will try to go beyond using the leads given in the biblical stories to help people create or interpret their own stories about working for business corporations. It will try to return the favor also by using the leads given in business stories to help believers understand their own stories about living faithfully in church.

Only when our storytelling is fully reciprocated, when the convergence envisioned involves mutual learning, will we be in a position to get full value from *Full Value*.

What Today's Business Stories May Tell Us

The argument presented so far is mostly theoretical. To test it, I should be able to frame an hypothesis about what one could expect to find in the stories told by businesspeople today, and then establish the signs of its plausibility. I have mentioned already the business narratives selected for this inquiry; what needs to be done now is to state clearly, based on my differences with Williams and Houck, what I expect these narratives to show that was not already evident in *Full Value*'s adaptation of Maccoby's *The Gamesman*. What I do not expect is to propose an alternative to Maccoby's typology, for the interpretation that I am hoping to develop may not be detachable from the narratives under examination. Placing these stories in a larger set of religious narratives is not meant to yield the kind of generalizations that Maccoby was after, namely, quasi-anthropological assertions claiming a scientific validity. Rather, the intent here is to improve our capacities for telling business stories by highlighting their unsuspected religious and theological dimensions. My hypothesis, therefore, is not that the religious dimension is unimportant, for surely it is, but that discerning it in business stories requires a theological perspective far more complex than the apparent dualism of Williams and Houck's "struggle to bring the values of the Kingdom of God into this world."

Of the four business narratives interpreted here, two are autobiographical and two are collective portraits drawn by business journalists. The autobiographical pieces, Michael Lewis's *Liar's Poker* and John H. Johnson's *Succeeding Against the Odds*, differ significantly from one another in that one is a *Bildungsroman* set, as the subtitle indicates, amid "the wreckage on Wall Street," while the other is a self-advertisement for "one of America's Wealthiest Entrepreneurs." What gives them significance in this context, however, is the resemblance between the story told by Lewis and *The Confessions* of St. Augustine insofar as both feature the moralizing recollections of an early philosophical retirement, and that of Johnson recalling *The Magnificat*, attributed to Mary the mother of Jesus, in that it celebrates the great reversal of fortune experienced by an oppressed poor person. Like Johnson's autobiography, Anne B. Fisher's portrait of *Wall Street Women* is a celebration of an oppressed group's new-found access to wealth and power. Though she and most of her informants probably would resist such an interpretation, her stories raise religious questions similar to those that liberation theology discovers in the Book of Exodus and the patterns of Deuteronomic history. Indeed, while each of these narratives is rich in moral passion, common to all three of them is the conventionally modern silence about God's activity in the world. Nevertheless, the resemblances with traditional religious narratives are striking, precisely because God's part has been so crudely cut out of them.

Michael Meyer's presentation of "the dreams that drive great businessmen" in *The Alexander Complex* is not so crude. In at least two of his portraits of Steven Jobs, Ross Perot, James Rouse, Robert Swanson, Ted Turner and Daniel Ludwig, God's activity is explicitly acknowledged by the entrepreneur under scrutiny. In all of them, the allusion to the heroic exploits of Alexander the Great ensures that God remains as significant a factor as He is in Hellenistic literature, symbolizing both the uncanny capriciousness of fortune and an inviolable limit to human aspiration and achievement. Though similar to Maccoby's project in its focus on the psychological relationship of personal character and work, Meyer's presentation is far more useful because it lacks serious commitment to the explanatory power of psychoanalysis. Some of the stories, notably Jobs' and Turner's, almost beg for clinical interpretation, yet Meyer is content to let the interviewees speak for themselves, with only modest intrusions of the leads given in the story of Alexander the Great.

Meyer's modesty, however, allows us to be bold. The collective portrait of *The Alexander Complex* calls for the mature Augustinian narrative of *The City of God*, in which the virtues of the noble Greeks and Romans are eulogized and then transcended in an apology for the Christian way of life. Just as St. Augustine's comic vision allows his readers to acknowledge that the strivings of the *civitas terrena* will continue to mingle with those of the *civitas Dei* until the Last Day, so we may be able to assist these modern Alexanders or, at least, their disciples, to discover the all too frequently ironic ways in which God finds a part for them in His own story. Unlike the young Augustine—and the precocious Michael Lewis—they will be able to discern that part, not in philosophical retirement, but through active engagement in a world whose moral ambiguity itself testifies to God's saving presence. As St.

Augustine himself would confess, Alexander's tragic failure is but a preparation for God's comic triumph in Jesus Christ.

But to begin at the beginning. Michael Lewis became a bond salesman for Salomon Brothers because, even among Princeton graduates, there were very few jobs for art history majors. From the start, he confesses that he was in it for the money. Yet only two years out of the Salomon Brothers training program, in January 1988 Lewis removed himself from their London offices, observing that "I thought it would be better to tell the story than to go on living the story."[19] The resulting narrative is about many things but mostly about unresolved moral conflict. Lewis is both fascinated and appalled by the Animal House atmosphere of the Salomon Brothers training program and the compellingly obnoxious culture of the floor traders. Indeed, he refrains wisely from excessive moralizing and admits, instead, his own need for acceptance by this group. Yet, in the end, once he has outgrown the greed that got him started on Wall Street, he could find no reason to stay in the business, and so he retires to his writer's cottage outside London.

Though much of his tale is quite critical of the firm, Lewis insists that the book is not motivated by any bitterness against Salomon Brothers. No less than the survivors of many another institutional bootcamp, Lewis displays the pride of one who enjoys being associated with an outfit regarded as the toughest and smartest on the Street. There are aspects of Salomon Brothers' corporate culture that he genuinely admires, mostly a fading code of loyalty, reflecting the firm's Jewish immigrant origins. Though this same ethos spawns some predictably raw, macho hazing rituals, Lewis recognizes both their importance in establishing these loyalties and their injustice to those excluded by them. His regrets, however, focus less upon the manner of the trials that he endured successfully than on the ways in which he came to use and abuse customers to further his own, and the firm's, objectives. Many a small investor was "blown up" by Lewis, as he learned through trial and error the subtleties of buying and selling bonds.

Writing from his philosophical retreat, Lewis now recognizes that his initiation at Salomon Brothers coincided with a near fatal transformation in the firm's ethos. The old system of tribal loyalties, informally governed by the firm's "rabbis," was breaking down because of the unprecedented expansion of activity on Wall Street during "the Roaring Eighties" and the defection of key people in the firm, who learned that, contrary to Salomon's traditionally hierarchical patterns of deferred compensation, they could cash in quickly on their momentary successes by switching to other, upstart firms like Drexel Burnham. For the best of Salomon's younger representatives "short term greed" seemed to be a more powerful motivator than traditional loyalties, and though Lewis exhibits a nostalgic fascination for the firm's traditions, he chafed against the firm's compensation policies also, at least until he had found it within himself to become detached from money making.

Lewis refuses to speculate on what shape Salomon Brothers' corporate ethos ought to take to survive the current contraction on Wall Street, but he does offer a few remarks on his own change of heart.

> I believe that I walked away from the clearest shot I'll ever have at being a millionaire....For me, however, the belief in the meaning of making dollars crumbled; the proposition that the more money you earn, the better the life you are leading was refuted by too much evidence to the contrary. And without that belief, I lost the need to make huge sums of money. The funny thing is that I was largely unaware how heavily influenced I was by the money belief until it had vanished.[20]

Lest we assume that he is contemplating a Franciscan vow of poverty, Lewis emphatically points out that he is living well off the serious money he made during his brief career and that, yes, he still holds stock in Salomon Brothers.

What is the religious dimension to Lewis's story? There is nothing concrete to suggest anything by way of religious convictions on his part, so our experiment is unconstrained by any allusions to religious narratives that Lewis might have woven into his story. I cannot help but read *Liar's Poker* in the perspective of *The Confessions* of St. Augustine, though Lewis's hindsight is hardly formed by the religious conversion and the necessities of pastoral office that shaped Augustine's account of his own early life.[21] Nevertheless, the two seem to intersect at a point prior to Augustine's conversion, perhaps, the Neoplatonic period in Milan when he agonized over abandoning his teaching career to pursue Christian wisdom. Like Lewis, Augustine was a young man on the make, who had overcome certain cultural barriers to full acceptance by his chosen peers. Major worldly success was at hand but he withdrew from it as he came to realize how empty of meaning it had actually become for him. Augustine's philosophical retirement, however, was soon to be ended after his conversion, for the Christian community of North Africa was virtually to kidnap him later into its pastoral service.

No one knows, of course, what God has yet in store for Michael Lewis. But from the perspective of *The Confessions,* he can be regarded, like the youthful Augustine, as another "natural man," whose depraved innocence is so thick that his most eloquent testimony regarding the redeeming presence of God can only be his sheer ignorance of Him. Lewis, like the natural man, is a decent fellow, the sort who sees withdrawal from the world as the only way to preserve his apparent integrity. On the other side of the kind of conversion Augustine experienced, such a withdrawal will come to be seen as an exquisitely pathetic form of self-indulgence. But Lewis does not yet know how to act responsibly in a world both steeped in sin and suffused by the grace of God, and so he sits on the sidelines and scribbles. Lewis's retirement is depressing for what it suggests about one young person's estimate of the prospects for business ethics, but any other view of the situation, it seems, can spring only from a faith far more robust than his.

In turning from *Liar's Poker* to John H. Johnson's *Succeeding Against the Odds,* we encounter the kind of faith that moves mountains: Johnson's faith in himself, his faith in the promise of the Afro-American community, and his faith in entrepreneurial capitalism. But is his a religious faith? Can it be placed in the context of Christian narrative? Johnson's book is clearly within the spectrum of inspirational literature extolling the virtues of business success. Its only claim to distinction is that its author is a self-affirming Afro-American who has overcome the stigma of racism and, in the process of almost singlehandedly organizing the economic potential of the Afro-American consumer market, has made himself the kingpin of a communications empire worth a quarter of a billion dollars. Johnson takes pride in his roots among the Afro-Americans of Arkansas City, Arkansas. Several times he returns to the story of how he got his start in the publishing business because his mother, Gertrude Johnson Williams, risked their only possessions, their furniture, as collateral on the $500 loan that launched *Negro Digest.* He is generous in acknowledging the boost he got from established Afro-American entrepreneurs in his adopted hometown of Chicago, and he glories in the recognition he has received, from the late fifties on, for championing the Civil Rights movement through his publications, including *Ebony.* So successful was Johnson's entrée into the overlapping political, cultural and corporate elites in this country that he came to be regarded as "Black America's special ambassador to White America."

Though Johnson clearly has learned to be at ease in these circles, his story never lets us forget that inside this epitome of Afro-American entrepreneurship still lives the youth who endured the indignities of the Jim Crow system of racial segregation. As Johnson sees it, he survived Jim Crow and rose to the challenges that his unprecedented success would bring, largely on the strength of a family and community life in which "every Black adult was charged with the responsibility of monitoring and supervising every Black child."[22] Not surprisingly, his story is filled with inspirational lessons on what blessings persistence, hard work, faith in one's own abilities, and a sharp eye on the main chance can bring. What otherwise might strike the reader as mere boastfulness is understood better as Johnson's continual attempt to convince himself that the stunning success he has become really did happen to him.

As I have indicated already, if there is a religious dimension to Johnson's story, he has chosen to keep it to himself. Though he mentions approvingly his mother's involvement in the Black church and his early fascination with the ministry, he tends to view the church primarily as an important social institution. The minister's power and prestige in the Afro-American community is what attracted him, though throughout his story he maintains an attitude of respectful acceptance, based primarily on the strength of his mother's faith. One of the few occasions where God enters this narrative is when Johnson tells of the tragic death of his adopted son, John, Jr., who battled sickle cell anemia for twenty-five years before succumbing to it:

> I've said many times that I believe the Lord sent him to our home so we could prolong his life. We suffered most of those twenty-five years and we were blessed in terms of what Gladys Knight called in her song, "the pain and glory"—because there was always pain, and yet there was always happiness and glory.[23]

The very casualness of the Lord's presence in this remark, coupled with the muted cadences of Black church rhetoric that have shaped Johnson's way of telling his story, suggest he may be on more intimate terms with God than he lets on in this book. Perhaps he and his collaborator, Lerone Bennett, Jr., felt that the conventions of business storytelling require the same sort of pretense of secularity that falsifies Bill Cosby's television portrayal of successful Afro-American family life. Or perhaps, the price of success for Johnson and Cosby involves an almost complete fade out of one's religious roots.

Were I to supply a Christian narrative against which Johnson's story might be retold, Mother Mary's *Magnificat* (Luke 1:46-55) might be an appropriate choice. This song of thanksgiving brings fresh focus to many scriptural themes from the Old Testament and seems especially dependent upon the song of Hannah (1 Samuel 2:1-10) which expresses the hope of "the poor of Yahweh." Its place in the infancy narrative of the Gospel of Luke helps reinforce not only the claim of Messiahship for Jesus, but also highlights Luke's interpretation of this claim as a vindication of the oppressed. It contains two leads that may be significant for interpreting Johnson's story, namely, the confession not only that it is the Almighty who has done these great things but also that His actions constitute a dramatic reversal of the world's own structures of power and domination. Great things have happened in Johnson's story, and Johnson himself certainly cherishes them as a turnaround that is significant not only for himself but for all Afro-Americans. But is it the Almighty who has done these things? If Johnson's faith in himself ultimately depends on recognizing God's own faithfulness, as it did for Hannah and Mary and their children, he is uncharacteristically shy about sharing this conviction with his readers.

What difference, if any, would it make for Johnson to have made of his story, like Mother Mary's *Magnificat*, a song of thanksgiving? Is there a way, in today's business world, to testify to God's saving power without sounding like a religious fanatic trying to convert the Almighty into some form of comparative advantage? If *The Magnificat* is to provide a plot for a certain range of business stories, the public character of its claim regarding God's activity in the world must be taken seriously, as well as the ambivalence that such a claim creates for both the recipients of Divine favor and their fellows who have not been so favored. Throughout the Bible and subsequent Jewish and Christian traditions, those blessed by God have had to struggle with the problem of "Election" or "Chosenness." Beginning with the story of Cain and Abel, the Bible recognizes that God's favor has been the occasion for jealousy and murderous resentment as well as thanksgiving. And yet if the truth of God's activity is to be recognized, that favor must be affirmed and celebrated in public. For, consistent with the Biblical perspective, God's favor is never merely a private benefit.

Any successful entrepreneur, like Johnson, whose business story needs to be sung as a chorus to the *Magnificat*, will have to learn the subtle art of communicating one's vision without excluding those who do not yet share in its blessings. The risk of alienating one's fellows by boasting of God's favor cannot be eliminated from business storytelling, any more than it has been eliminated from the traditions of biblical narrative. Yet, at least in this particular case, Johnson seems to be a master of the subtle art of inclusiveness, for he has been enormously successful in persuading the elites of White America that they have nothing to lose and everything to gain from the political and economic advancement of Black America. What he has learned by successfully marketing Afro-American culture challenges all Christians to communicate the story of our common religious destiny more effectively. Were Johnson to see his own story in terms of the *Magnificat*, he would be the first to insist that God's favor cannot be a zero-sum game.

Johnson's optimistic faith in himself and in the Afro-American community finds an impressive, though less impassioned parallel in Anne B. Fisher's *Wall Street Women*. Hers is a collective portrait of the first generation of women to be making a significant impact on the folkways of the investment industry. The scale of this shy revolution is impressive: During the 15-year period from 1972 to 1987, the percentage of women in professional positions on Wall Street "increased fivefold to just over 25 percent, and the proportion was still rising."[24] To get some handle on what this figure means, Fisher points out that according to the American Economic Association, within the ranks of academia, "only 3 to 4 percent of all full professors were female in both 1975 and 1985," though over the same period the number of PhDs in economics earned by women increased from 11 to 18 percent.[25] The dramatic changes in the composition of Wall Street's labor force raises a question that Fisher and her informants are exploring actively, namely, whether women can be expected to transform the corporate cultures of Wall Street, or be absorbed by them. The results of her inquiries, not surprisingly, are mixed.

One of the most intriguing metaphors offered by one of her informants compares women's recent gains on Wall Street to familiar immigrant stories. Susan Byrne, who founded Westwood Management, has created a different kind of corporate culture by hiring an almost exclusively female staff for her firm.

> "I get teased sometimes for having an attitude like an immigrant," Susan remarks. "Because one thing immigrants always do is, once the first one gets established, he brings in the next one, and the next one, and the next one, and the next, and the next....Well, Wall Street has

always welcomed immigrants. First came the Jews, then the Irish, then Italians, and now women. So, if you look at it that way, women coming to Wall Street, and helping other women to get ahead too, is just the latest expansion of a very old pattern."[26]

Without placing too fine a point on it, Fisher's account seems to take this observation as a lead into the Wall Street women's stories, for she tends to assume that their thinking and acting will be animated by a common ethnic culture, the shape of which it is her task to discern.

There are perhaps three salient features to this women's culture on Wall Street, and each of these may turn out to be a comparative advantage for business success during the 1990s. First, though women have demonstrated themselves to be just as competent as men in the invest-ment industry, their work histories are far more diverse. Many of the women are embarked upon second careers after having been oriented earlier in life toward the so-called helping professions. Second, the women interviewed by Fisher seem to have a different attitude toward making money from that typically exhibited by the men. In a way that corroborates Michael Lewis's observations, Fisher analyzes "Trader Head,...the macho habit of equating money with self-esteem."[27] While admittedly women do occasionally suffer from this malady, she reports the observation of Leslie Daniels who explains: "Women don't define their entire existence by how much they make. What money does buy, for us, is not self-acceptance—which we tend to get from other sources— but *security*.[28] Third, women are less likely to succumb to the oppressive syndrome of workaholism that became fashionable during the 'Roaring Eighties.' " Characterizing Wall Street since the late seventies as "a kind of mercenary monastery, a haven for the bright but socially malad-justed,"[29] Fisher observes how women are giving each other permission to seek and express a sense of balance in their lives through serious attention to a variety of private and public activities, ranging from *pro bono* work organizing a shelter for battered women to raising a family.

In the aftermath of the stock market collapse of October 1987, it became fashionable, as Fisher notes, for both men and women to question the dominant Wall Street ethos. After the Crash, the cavalier attitudes toward customers that Michael Lewis had denounced quickly came to be regarded as counterproductive as investors abandoned Wall Street for less risky and less predatory ventures. What some have viewed as the ensuing "Return to Normalcy" in the financial markets is likely to favor the advancement of women, as Fisher sees it, for their distinctive cultural background is more naturally oriented toward serving the needs of others than was the ferociously competitive ethos that is passing. Fisher's story thus is a remarkably understated celebration of a people's emergent triumph, the story of an immigration that so far promises not to end in the excesses of overweening pride and domination. Her story is a hopeful one, remarkably lacking in anger or a sense of grievance. It suggests that if women on Wall Street maintain the solidarity forced originally upon them by circumstances, they may be able to have a transformative impact on how all of us conduct business in this country.

If there is a religious dimension to the story of this latter day immigrant group, it does not surface in Fisher's account. Even in the chapter narrating "The Search for Balance," religion enters only to the extent that one of her informants, Karen Robards, founded the Cooke School for Special Education which is affiliated with the Roman Catholic Archdiocese of New York.[30] Without further instruction from her, we must assume that Wall Street women find churches no more than occasionally useful as institutional underwriters of some of their good works. But perhaps we are looking for religiousness in the wrong places. Perhaps Fisher's informants do not equate religion with active church membership but, say, with direct personal encounters with nature. Fisher's retelling of Sarah Boehmler's story of her Outward Bound expedition into the wilderness offers ample opportunity but no direct evidence of religious experience. If anything, nature is not an occasion for aesthetic contemplation but for Sarah, at least, another opportunity to demonstrate a competitive spirit, not at all dissimilar to the daily challenge of coping with the pressures of Wall Street. So, once again, we are left to our own speculations. What sort of religious narrative might provide the ultimate framework for interpreting Fisher's shy revolution?

Because Fisher's is the collective portrait of a group's movement from the periphery to the center of business activity, a movement that is triumphing over societal marginalization, my choice is the biblical narrative of Exodus, particularly as it gives rise to the Deuteronomic pattern of historical interpretation. The focus of this narrative, of course, is Israel, the People of God, and how God acted to change the course of history by making a covenant with them. Though the story does recall Israel's oppression in Egypt, its central theme is the exercise of public responsibility. If Israel is to prosper as a People, enjoying the fruits of God's favor in the Promised Land, it must remain faithful to the covenant. Faithful obedience is the key to preserving the meaning of its liberation. Deuteronomic history, it seems, is an attempt to make sense of what actually happened to the People of God, an accounting of Israel's stewardship in the Promised Land, in light of this simple proposition. When Israel was successful in conquering its enemies and in reorganizing the resources of the Promised Land for its own life, its success was attributed to the leadership's faithfulness, and the root of its eventual failure, to their faithlessness. In either event, God's sovereignty was magnified.

If Fisher's women wish to fancy themselves as an immigrant group on Wall Street, they would do well to consider the bittersweet experience of the original People of God, for the parallels are obvious. Fisher and her informants know, just as Israel came to recognize, that the constellation of events that occasioned their liberation are beyond their control, as are the dramatic shifts in market forces that may allow Wall Street women to become the pacesetters in the investment industry for the 1990s and beyond. She implies also that, for their success to be meaningful, it must mean something more than simply getting a fair share of the rewards of money making. Though that something more remains unnamed by Fisher, the stories Wall Street women tell about themselves suggest a commitment to service, an ethic of stewardship, and a corporate culture in which community is not just another slogan.

When it comes to explaining how these transformative possibilities exist within this particular group of immigrants, however, Fisher falls back upon truisms asserting the distinctiveness of women's experience. Yet these assertions seem empty in light of the stories her informants tell, stories that offer little hope that, as the number of women on Wall Street continues to increase, their actions will still exhibit the solidarity of an immigrant group. Once that solidarity disappears, there is every reason to think that the transformative possibilities will tend to evaporate as well. Viewed in the perspective of Deuteronomic history, the story of women on Wall Street is not yet that of a People. They remain suspended on the threshold of history for lack of a covenant with God.

"Without vision, the People perish!" warns at least one countercultural bumper sticker. Will logic permit us to have faith in ourselves and our fellows, without anchoring that faith in some larger vision of the human enterprise? Must the entrepreneur's personal vision be shared if the transformative possibilities implicit in it are to be realized? Michael Meyer's study, *The Alexander Complex*, more than any of the narratives considered so far, confronts these theological questions and answers them affirmatively. The narrative, however, remains in the noncommittal mode of tragic irony because, as the title suggests, the fate of Alexander the Great awaits even the most ambitious of these business people. Meyer makes no attempt to establish the relative adequacy of the various visions presented, apart from describing their psychological consequences for the visionaries who hold them. So Steven Jobs's obsession with his own genius, and his demand that his followers demonstrate an almost Messianic faith in his leadership, is on a par not only with the apocalyptic fantasies that prompted Ted Turner to found the Better World Society but also with developer James Rouse's Christian commitment to eliminating the problem of homelessness through his Enterprise Foundation. The ironic parallels with the career of Alexander the Great reach a climax in the final chapter where we witness Daniel Ludwig squander perhaps a billion dollars on the futile dream of carving out a jungle kingdom for himself in the Amazon basin of Brazil. As the visionary ends up metaphorically blinding himself to his own limitations, Meyer leaves us to contemplate the Alexandrine *hubris* of a "complex" that fittingly "should contain the seed of self-destruction."[31]

People perish for lack of vision but, as Meyer implies, they may also perish precisely because of it. We leave Meyer's narrative wondering what God can be, if human aspiration and achievement, especially when animated by such large visions, inevitably must end in futility. In such a narrative, God may be a symbol for the power of "Creative Destruction" that Schumpeter identified with the marketplace. We honor this god when we get caught up in the Whirlwind of its transformative activity, knowing full well—at least by the time it is through with us—that it will destroy us. True to the classic tradition of Greek tragedy, Meyer does not advocate that we abandon the stage in favor of philosophical retirement; instead, he implies that we should accept our fate and play our roles with only the consolation of having been touched by a great adventure.

Unquestionably, Meyer's is a religious narrative but, unlike the other stories we have considered, this one raises the question as to whether the religiousness conveyed here is true religion. Is Meyer's God the true God? A Christian theologian's answer to this question would hardly be surprising but, perhaps, the manner of approaching the question could be. Consistent with the general assumptions of narrative theology, the only response to a defective religious narrative is to provide a better one.

The issues raised by *The Alexander Complex*, I am suggesting, are appropriately considered in the context of St. Augustine's monumental opus, *The City of God*, for here the religious stories of the Greeks and Romans, including the tragedies, are criticized and reconstructed as part of the Christian story. Though Augustine offers the definitive apology for Latin Christianity, the question animating his narrative he shares with his Greek and Roman antagonists: how God acts in history, and with what consequences for understanding ourselves, our aspirations and achievements. Augustine rejects the idea of Fate expressed in the tragic vision presupposed by *The Alexander Complex*, and affirms a Christian faith in Divine Providence or the Will of God. As Augustine's own manner of discourse in *The City of God* suggests, the difference between the two can be grasped only in narrative.

It is the Will of God that human aspiration and achievement be not in vain. Though the worship of Fate feigns a submission to the Will of God, it actually yields only what Meyer drew from it, namely, the contemplation of the lessons of *hubris* which eventually tempt us either to philosophical detachment or to an undiscerning acceptance of the world as it is. Augustine's vision in *The City of God* tries to contrast tragedy with comedy while retaining an indispensably humanizing touch of irony.[32] Keeping faith with the Will of God means relying upon God's promises, within which the whole of human history is implicated. Christian faith affirms the meaningfulness of human aspiration and achievement, not necessarily on their own terms, but in terms of God's saving purposes. Faith in Divine Providence rests upon a recognition of the inextricable way in which all human enterprises, symbolized by the *civitas terrena*, contribute toward building up the eternal *civitas Dei*. As a result, Augustine would not agree with Meyer's verdict on the Alexander Complex but, consistent with his ironic recognition of the virtues of the noble Greeks and Romans, would praise the achievements of Meyer's great businessmen while seeking to refine, and eventually transform, their ultimate aspirations. Noble enterprises need not end in futility if they serve a purpose higher than human glory. That purpose is the story of the City of God.

The Role of Religious Narrative in Business Ethics

I have tried to show in retelling these four stories that the role of narrative in business ethics need not be restricted to questions of character formation, nor does the Christian story necessarily require a confrontational attitude toward the routine procedures of business corporations. The fact is that businesses, like other human organizations, already tend to live and die by the stories that are told in them. No apology for narrative as such is needed, but perhaps greater discernment is. The result need not be a typology or any other set of moralizing abstractions. On the contrary, refining the business of storytelling in business means learning to extend the stories told by businesspeople in ways that make their religious implications inescapably evident.

If the narratives analyzed here are at all representative, the stories told by businesspeople raise issues that will require theologians and ethicists to broaden their own horizons. Those committed to genuine listening will be forced to focus on the central questions regarding the mystery of God's activity among us, and the evidence for it in the patterns of our daily activity as individuals and within institutions. Discernment will require setting aside conventional preoccupations with moral quandaries, to renew the search for those ultimate meanings that animate our common enterprises. It will challenge us also to be bold in affirming the breadth and depth of religiousness in the United States, despite the secularity evident in most business narratives, to overcome what seems to be a powerful literary convention forbidding any acknowledgement of God's part in business stories.

This chapter, however, has not been limited to these methodological points. I have tried to suggest also the relevance of a particular theological perspective, that of classical Christian theology, the perspective of the Divine Comedy celebrated by Dante, systematized by Aquinas and envisioned by Augustine. This perspective, I believe, still contains unique resources for coping with the moral ambiguities involved in accepting managerial responsibility within a world that already, at least partially, reflects the impact of centuries of Christian witness. Other theologians who have recognized the importance of religious narrative have tended to emphasize the confrontational message of the New Testament. Although I have no desire to water down the Gospel, I think we run the risk of falsifying our situation if we pretend that we respond to its message in ignorance of nearly two millennia of Christian tradition that can still instruct us regarding the ambiguities of faithfulness in this world. Such a substantive claim can hardly be made persuasively with just a handful of allusions to *The City of God*, but I hope to have shown enough here to make it worth pursuing.

Notes

1. The contributions of Hauerwas and MacIntyre to programs of theological ethics responsive to the narrative traditions of the Christian communities are situated nicely within the larger discussion of this field in the recent volume edited by Hauerwas and L. Gregory Jones, *Why Narrative? Readings in Narrative Theology* (Grand Rapids, MI: Eerdmans Publishing Co., 1989).

2. Alasdair MacIntyre, *After Virtue* (Notre Dame, IN: University of Notre Dame Press, 1981).

3. Stanley Hauerwas, *The Peaceable Kingdom: A Primer in Christian Ethics* (Notre Dame, IN: University of Notre Dame Press, 1983).

4. Oliver F. Williams and John W. Houck, *Full Value: Cases in Christian Business Ethics* (San Francisco: Harper and Row, 1978).

5. The inadequacies of business ethics programs based on "the standard account of morality" are well aired in my essay, "Religious Studies and Business Ethics: New Directions in an Emerging Field," *The Journal of Business Ethics*, vol. 5. No. 6 (December 1986). I served as editor for this symposium.

6. Michael Maccoby, *The Gamesman: The New Corporate Leaders* (New York, NY: Simon and Schuster, 1976).

7. Michael Lewis, *Liar's Poker: Rising Through the Wreckage on Wall Street* (New York, NY: W.W. Norton, 1989).

8. John H. Johnson with Lerone Bennett, Jr., *Succeeding Against the Odds: The Inspiring Autobiography of One of America's Wealthiest Entrepreneurs* (New York, NY: Warner Books, 1989).

9. Michael Meyer, *The Alexander Complex* (New York, NY: Times Books/ Random House, 1989).

10. Anne B. Fisher, *Wall Street Women: Women in Power on Wall Street Today* (New York, NY: Alfred A. Knopf, 1989).

11. Williams and Houck, p. 38.

12. *Ibid.*, p. 24.

13. *Ibid.*, p. 42.

14. Maccoby, 1976.

15. Williams and Houck, p. 74, footnote 13.

16. *Ibid.*, pp. 61-67.

17. *Ibid.*, p. 61.

18. An appropriately theological understanding of business corporations was outlined in passing by James M. Gustafson and Elmer W. Johnson in their essay, "The Corporate Leader and the Ethical Resources of Religion: A Dialogue," in the volume edited by Houck and Williams, *The Judeo-Christian Vision and the Modern Corporation* (Notre Dame, IN: University of Notre Dame Press, 1982). Gustafson and Johnson describe corporations as aspects

of "divine governance" in the world. This term allows them a role in the full panoply of God's activity, while also respecting the ecclesiological distinction between them and the Christian churches.

19. Lewis, p. 9.

20. *Ibid.*, p. 248.

21. The choice of St. Augustine's *Confessions* is not an arbitrary one, but is suggested by the similarities of literary form and by the constitutive role of Augustine's thinking in defining the theological horizon that I am attempting to demonstrate here. This convergence of literary and theological considerations will govern the selections made throughout this section of the chapter. My views of Augustine and his works are mostly in accord with those expressed by the historian Peter Brown in his acclaimed study, *Augustine of Hippo, A Biography* (Berkeley: University of California Press, 1967).

22. Lewis, p. 37.

23. *Ibid.*, p. 256.

24. Fisher, p. 59.

25. *Ibid.*, p. 127.

26. *Ibid.*, p. 75.

27. *Ibid.*, p. 89.

28. *Ibid.*, p. 91.

29. *Ibid.*, p. 147.

30. *Ibid.*, p. 164.

31. Meyer, p. 249.

32. The significance of irony in historial interpretation is widely recognized by modern theologians, beginning with Reinhold Niebuhr's seminal work, *The Irony of American History* (New York: Charles Scribner's Sons, 1952), and is the organizing theme in Martin E. Marty's recent work, *Modern American Religion: Volume I: The Irony of It All (1893-1919)* (Chicago, IL: University of Chicago Press, 1986). The Augustinian background of this perspective is discussed briefly in my essay, "What's So Christian About Christian Realism?" *The Bible in American Law, Politics and Rhetoric*, ed. James T. Johnson (Philadelphia, PA: Fortress Press, 1984), which shows that irony is what distinguishes Niebuhr's political philosophy from that of other Cold War realists like Hans Morgenthau.

Nine

The Moral Theology of Silas Lapham

Thomas L. Shaffer

> Our manners and customs go for more in life than our qualities. The price we pay for civilization is the fine yet impassable differentiation of these. Perhaps we pay too much; but it will not be possible to persuade those who have the difference in their favor that this is so.

William Dean Howells

Story

What you need for the study of virtue in business is the story of a good person who is in business. Silas Lapham, the titular hero of William Dean Howells's novel about American business in the so-called Gilded Age, was such a good person. He was what was then called a gentleman; he was what Aristotle called a man of practical wisdom; in Yiddish, he was a *mensch*.

It is not remarkable that a novelist of the American realist school was interested in good people at work; we have many such stories about doctors, lawyers, and even politicians. A nineteenth-century story about a good person in *business* is not remarkable either. I think of Thomas Mann's *Buddenbrooks* or the George Eliot or Anthony Trollope characters who were, as the Victorians put it, "in trade" (Adam Bede is an example, as is the remarkable woman who married Dr. Thorne, Miss Dunstable.) R.F. Delderfield has at least two trilogies about British business families in the nineteenth century, and then there are all those Forsytes.

But it is unusual to find a story about someone who is a good person, in business, in the United States. Our culture, which has produced more sustained business success than any other, and which has distributed the benefits of business more widely than any other, has produced almost no business hero stories. If you consult only our stories you will decide that our business people are self-deceived or rapacious, or both. Sinclair Lewis's George F. Babbitt is at one end of the spectrum; Arthur Miller's Joe Keller is at the other; J.P. Marquand's sincere Willis Wade is in the middle. Our most popular stories of good people in business are stories of exit: The hero is a hero because he got out in time; Gregory Peck as "The Man in the Gray Flannel Suit" and William Holden in "Executive Suite" are examples. These stories say that business is no place for a person with a conscience.

Which means something is skewed. The value of stories in ethics is that they give access to common sense with relatively little interference from concepts. Common sense says that business in the United States is not corrupting, even if business stories say it is. We know good people in business. Some of them are in *big* business. They live next door to us; we worship with them; we get wise advice from them as we buy our cough medicine and hardware. They are our parents and our children, our sisters, brothers, aunts and uncles. They are our friends, and friendship, Aristotle says, is collaboration in the good.

The problem, I suspect, is that our popular stories about business are not in touch with reality. Post-war (World War II) stories such as Sloan Wilson's *The Man in the Gray Flannel Suit* and Cameron Hawley's *Executive Suite* portray business life as tragedy. Howells, the realist, was interested in the ordinary in business life. He said tragedy was useless to him, because tragedy obscures character: "It stuns all the faculties, all the emotions except a single one—defiance....[C]haracter is passive under the weight it cannot lift or shift or move," he said. "Man is a creature of light; tragedy is darkness....The study of human character is best pursued in the normal daily round, with its...ills for which it ever has its uses and its cures."

The issue is what is truthful. Wilson and Hawley wrote business stories that are tragic and, therefore, not useful; they are not useful because they are not true. Defiance would have been the morally appropriate response to the U.S. business world as they described it, but the choice they gave, between business and sound morals, is not the way life is. Elaine Hedges, a perceptive critic, calls it "mid-Victorian." She means these stories are romantic, tragic and forced—and *not true*.

Business is crippled in finding solutions for its ethical issues if we do not have truthful business stories to tell and to hear, and we academics are crippled in finding issues for our ethical solutions. We need truthful stories. We listen to stories to find out the issues. When I think I have learned what the issues are, and then their appropriate answers, I go back to the story to see if I am right. The story is my *epistemology*. We need storytellers so we can know, and we need them so we know that we know.

Analytical Structure

I approach the business story I am going to work on here, when I get around to it, as Aristotle approached the man of practical wisdom: I go to the story knowing that the person who acts in it is a good person. What I want to know is how this person goes about being good in business. What are the ethical issues for him or her? And what does he or she do with them? What are the moral rules? And how does this person live with these moral rules?

If this Aristotelian structure is useful, the story will respond to an inquiry about virtue in business in four ways:[1]

1. It will describe virtue as the *middle way*. Aristotle said that the virtue of courage is the middle way between cowardice and recklessness, for example. Cowardice is a deficiency of courage; recklessness is an excess of it. He tested his perception of virtue by locating the extremes: The moral way is in the middle.

2. The story will describe virtues in business in reference to the *goal* of a life in business. Life is a journey; journeys are pointed somewhere, and virtues are what help us along the way, as vices are what hold us back.

3. The story will describe virtue as *skill*, as moral craftsmanship, rather like craftsmanship in management, finance, accounting or marketing. We do not come to be virtuous because we survive ominous moral testing or choose right when stakes are high. We survive, if we do, because we are virtuous; but we come to be virtuous, or not, because of what we do on ordinary Wednesday afternoons in small matters. We are trained in virtue; it is something we learn from teachers. Virtue is habit and discipline; we study it as we might study how to make pots. The story that tells me about virtue in business

will tell me what the moral skills in business are, and it will show me the teachers.

4. The story will *tell the truth* about life as it tries to tell me what is virtuous in life. The romantic, tragic American business story fails at this because it shows too little of business life, too little of the ills of the normal daily round, for which character ever has its uses and its cures. It fails at truthfulness because it exaggerates the weight of moral choice.

The tragic and romantic business stories are relatively useless for an Aristotelian story method for an additional reason: They depend on the distinction between fact and value. They are like cases in an appellate court, where conscience as judge considers the "facts of a case" and then pronounces a judgment based on principles. Aristotelian (and, in this case, Platonic and Socratic) method insists that the ways we perceive and relate to what is going on around us, and the way we describe what has gone on around us, are as much exercises of virtue and vice as the way we decide what to do. Perception, relation and description *are* the way we decide what to do. "Seeing is a moral art," as Iris Murdoch puts it. Truthful description is the exercise of virtue. Disaster in the moral lives of people who work is not the decision to be evil; it is self-deception, as self-deception is the disaster behind the disaster in tragic American business stories.

My favorite American business story is Howells's *The Rise of Silas Lapham.* I propose to discuss it in the following four Aristotelian ways.

Virtue as the Middle Way

Silas was one of several children of a farm family in Vermont. He grew up on the farm and married the village school teacher whose name was Persis. They had a son who died when a child and two daughters, Penelope and Irene. His business was the manufacture and distribution of a "noninflammable" mineral paint. The mineral for the paint came from a vein his father found when the wind blew over an old tree on the farm.

Silas did not decide at first to be a paint magnate. He was a farmer. "All my brothers went West," he said, "and took up land; but I hung on to New England, and I hung on to the old farm, not because the paint mine was on it, but because the old house was—and the graves."

He returned to the farm after service in the Civil War, but he worked also in town to get enough money to do something with his unusual natural resource. He sacrificed, as an entrepreneur does in the American dream, to build a "works" on the farm for boiling the mineral in linseed oil and packaging it as paint. The business grew; the paint was marketed nationally. Silas opened an office in Boston; he, Persis, Penelope and Irene, still rural Vermonters, found themselves in a lavish but not fashionable house in Boston, with more money than they knew how to spend.

The story is about the relationship between two series of events. First, the Laphams made a run at Boston society, built a house in Back Bay that was fashionable as well as lavish, and began to trade calling cards and dinner invitations with the effete, old and respected Boston family of Bromfield Corey. Second, the business declined all the way into liquidation and Silas had to give up everything but his original "works." At the end of the story, the family has moved back to Lapham, Vermont, and Silas has returned to the simple, local business management of his early days. He boasts less in Vermont; he comes to look on his life in Boston more the way Puritans look on life in general. "Seems sometimes as if it was a hole opened for me," he says, "and I crept out of it."

The way Silas looked at his story reminded me of my friend Harry, a modern Puritan. Harry is a minister in the southern branch of the Presbyterian Church. His wife, referring to Harry's durable Calvinism, once defined his theology as a story. In the story she imagined, Harry tripped over the rug and fell down the stairs—head over heels, bump-bump-bump, all the way down. He lay there and rested a minute, then got up, brushed himself off, and said, "I'm glad that's over."

We could use, instead of Silas's own account, the way Sloan Wilson and Cameron Hawley looked at U.S. business in the prosperous years after World War II: "Business corrupts," they said. That might be useful, if it were true. It would say that Silas made a run at Boston, but he failed because he was a good man and would not be corrupted. Jan Dietrichson's critical study argues that as the meaning of Silas Lapham's story. It is the romantic-tragic reading that I do not find persuasive.

Another way to get at the ethics in Silas's story would be to say, as one study of Howells's novels does, that Silas is the "coarse soul" in a sophisticated business and social world: He fails because he does not have the urbane craftsmanship he needs for success in Boston. He is too simple for success in business and too unsubtle for success in society. This argument shares with Dietrichson's romantic-tragic "image of money" argument the perception that Silas needed to be in Vermont so he could be virtuous, but it differs in that it does not need to claim that the urban business and social worlds are corrupt. As Persis put it, discussing Bromfield Corey with Silas, "[I]t isn't what you've got, and it isn't what you've done, exactly. It's what you are." And *where* you are. Howells invited such an analysis when he said that the country had the advantage of creativity; cities, he said, are activity rather than substance. "I think we shall in time learn to do without cities," he said.

The second way of looking at the story says that business is gnostic rather than corrupt. Silas lacked the skills for coping with business. He was in the wrong place, and context matters. This was a prominent view of the novel among contemporary reviewers (H.E. Scudder for example), some of whom thought that Howells's novel portrayed Silas and Persis as more intelligent and sensitive than Vermont country people could possibly have been. These reviewers lived in cities.

There is an Aristotelian middle way between the tragic-romantic argument that American business is corrupt, and the gnostic view of it. Description of the middle way will require that I make a couple of distinctions. (The medieval Scholastics were Aristotelians, or at any rate Catholics, when they said, "Never deny; seldom affirm; always distinguish.")

The middle way says that what is important is how a person of character deals with circumstances. The circumstance in Silas's story was not a catastrophe that tested his moral fiber. It was the sort of thing with which any businessperson has to be able to deal: Some people in West Virginia discovered a mineral-paint mine down there. They built their own "works," and had the happy circumstance of cheap natural gas nearby. They could make paint as good as Lapham's, and for a lower price. This was neither a tragedy nor a mystery. It was a circumstance.

The ethical lessons, as Howells teaches them, have to do with how a good person handles circumstances today that are not as happy for him or her as were the circumstances of yesterday. The ethical argument Howells makes is that the skills a good person uses in the unhappy circumstance are the same skills used when times were better. The individual responds now, as then, with integrity, demonstrating character. Misfortune does not change the person into somebody else.

If integrity were important and if character were the focus, it makes no sense to read the story in the romantic, tragic, mid-Victorian way. It makes no sense to say that Silas's goodness is what built the business, and that his failure to be evil is what ruined it. Silas used the same moral skills, and Persis stood by his side, goading, teaching and supporting him in the same way when times were good as when times were bad. What you would have to do to sustain the business-corrupts argument is show why the moral skills with which they built the business did not work for them in keeping the business.

The plausibility of the mid-Victorian argument is that Silas might have succeeded if he had been willing to lie and cheat; but it would be as plausible to say that the reason Silas failed was that he did not rob a bank to cover his business losses. Not robbing banks served him well while the business grew but it stopped serving him well when he needed money, and so business survival would have corrupted him because business survival requires that you get money from robbery if you want to survive. That position is what Aristotle would have called excessive.

The other extreme is the "coarse soul" argument. It treats Silas as if he were uninitiated; it makes his business failure a failure of credentials, of priesthood. It is what Aristotle would have called deficient. The argument is not a plausible construction of the narrative because it overlooks two aspects of the story that the storyteller was bent on emphasizing—first, that Silas was a skillful business manager; even in Boston he was hailed in the press as "an example of single-minded application and unwavering perseverance which our young businessmen would do well to emulate." And, second, the gate-keepers of Boston society were entirely willing to admit rural Vermonters to their number if the Vermonters were willing to spend enough money. If what Silas needed was the approval of those who had and who could teach him the rituals of urban business success, he had only to buy what he needed. "Money buys position at once," Bromfield Corey says. "The world knows...how to drive a bargain....Well, then, they must spend. There is no other way for them to win their way to general regard."

The Aristotelian middle way is not a priesthood. It is the way of ordinary business skill. It is illustrated in the story by Tom Corey, Bromfield's son, who has inherited a Bostonian silver spoon, who courts the Lapham daughters, and who goes into Silas's company as a marketing manager. Tom has access to whatever status and urban skill Silas lacked. He has also enough wealth from his family to live well without going into trade, and is, therefore, a character Howells could have used to support the romantic-tragic, business-corrupts, mid-Victorian argument, if he had wanted to make it.

Tom wants to be a businessman; he wants to work in business as another well-heeled young man of his time and place might have wanted to explore the Amazon or study Sanskrit. Early in the story, when Tom has caught the eye of Irene Lapham, Silas disapproves of him on Puritan theological principle: "I don't see how a fellow like that...can hang 'round home and let his father support him. Seems to me, if I had his health and his education, I should want to strike out and do something for myself.... I like to see a man *act* like a man."

Silas changed his mind because Tom was serious about wanting to work in business. Then Silas says of Tom—and he is right, as things turn out—"He's a natural-born businessman.... I've had many a fellow with me that...worked hard all his life, without ever losing his original opposition to the thing. But Corey likes it."

The middle way sees business as something worthwhile to do. Something less than "Oedipus Rex," something more than a pirouette. Tom Corey is a focus for the point because he practices business when he does not need the money. His work in the paint business is a theater for the exercise of skill, *including moral skill.* Business, in Tom's anticipation, and, I think, in Howells's description, is what Alasdair MacIntyre calls a *practice.* The good of it is internal to the activity. It is done in significant part for its own sake. And that means that it is, or can be, according to MacIntyre's account, a school for the virtues of truthfulness, justice and courage. It is a way to become and to be a good person.

The view that outcomes in business are tragic, because virtue is not consistent with success in business, shares with this middle-way argument the perception that business is absorbing, that business beckons its people to serious involvement. The tragic view of business is, however, excessive. The view that business requires esoteric skills or credentials or recommendations that are not available to straightforward people shares with the middle-way argument the understanding that business is subtle. But the esoteric-skills position does not allow for the possibility that business will yield to clear motives and the energy of ordinary people.[2]

"I believe in my paint," Silas says. "I believe it's a blessing to the world." Although he, like most people in U.S. business, seems to lack the language for explaining the point, Silas is not in the paint business for the money. His belief in what he does is as transparent as it seems to be:

"You've got to believe in a thing before you can put any heart in it," he says. He does not mention wealth as a goal, nor manners as providing access to what he wants to do. Silas likes and then trusts Tom Corey because he senses in him the same interest in *doing* and the same willingness to believe that what he does is worthwhile. That is the middle way. It is excessive to equate business with money; it is deficient to equate business with manners; it is sensible and realistic to see business as something worthwhile to do.

Virtue and Goal

The difference between a business ethic of virtue and a business ethic of honor is that virtue depends on a goal—what the Aristotelians call a *teleology*—and honor depends on approval. There are businesspeople in Silas's story who fashion their morals according to what their peers approve of; theirs is an ethic of honor (when they get approval) and shame (when they do not).

Honor is not a particularly evil morality. The Aristotelian argument is that it is not an adequate morality. For example, Silas declined Tom Corey's investment in the business at a time when the business needed capital more than anything. But Silas thought the investment was too risky. Boston businessmen who found out what Silas had done considered the matter and announced that it was a gentlemanly, honorable thing to do; they nodded their heads and approved of it. The morality of honor and the morality of virtue coincided in that case.

Silas's behavior shows how the morality of the honorable gentleman had powerful force in Howells's day; it still does. The ordinary, mundane problem with it is its vulnerability to self-deception.[3] An example in this story is the amount of candor honor required when Silas's manufacturing business was courting investors.

Silas's response to the West Virginia competition was to negotiate a merger of the two enterprises; he sought to make the competition his own and in that way eliminate it. The deal he made gave him a week to raise the money to buy out the West Virginians. An investor came his way, an investor who knew that the Lapham company had been successful but did not know about the competition in West Virginia. The consensus among honorable businessmen was the market morality of *caveat emptor*—let the buyer beware. All that honor required was that a gentleman not lie. It was up to the investor to know what he was doing.

Caveat emptor had many defenders, most of whom talked about the importance of vigilance for worldly success. Some of them talked about the survival of the fittest.

Silas would not have been considered *dishonorable* if he had said nothing to his investor about the West Virginians. But he acted beyond what honor required of him, told the investor, and lost the deal. The poignant thing about the way Silas behaved in this episode, and in others involving investors—the thing that shows how honor works—is that he was candid with investors but he did not want anyone in the Boston business world to know he was. "He believed that he had acted right...and he was satisfied," Howells says, "but he did not care to have...anybody think he had been a fool." Silas knew about *caveat emptor* and the morals of honor; he respected the morals of honor; he knew those morals would protect him from censure if he followed *caveat emptor*. In the case of Tom Corey's proposed investment, Silas was pleased that the business gentlemen of Boston found him honorable. But honor was not his ethic; virtue was his ethic.

John Henry Newman said that, as admirable as he was, the nineteenth-century Christian gentleman finally could not cope with reality. It was not that the gentleman's morality was evil; it was that it could not deal with the depth and complexity of the evil around it. "You might as well moor your vessel with a thread of silk," Newman said, "or quarry granite with a razor." The morality of the Christian gentleman was not dependably Christian (or Jewish); it was, in Philip Mason's phrase, only a sub-cult of our Hebraic moral heritage. Its failure was precisely on Newman's point: It could not bear the truth of a moral tradition in which Israel suffers to overcome evil, and Jesus is tortured to death in the name of the law.

The more analytical criticism of the ethics of honor is that honor is not a virtue. Aristotle said, "[H]onor seems to depend on those who confer it rather than on him who receives it, whereas our guess is that the good is a person's own possession which cannot easily be taken away from him." The relevant virtue, he said, is not honor, but high-mindedness, a good habit that is the middle way between the excess of vanity and the deficiency of disdain for the approval of good people.

Virtue as Skill

Persis, the village school teacher, was Silas's Aristotelian master in the virtues, but she was also a Puritan and she made mistakes an English gentleman or an Athenian man of practical wisdom would not have made. One of the things we learn from stories is that moral masters are interesting people. They are not lecturers at podiums or writers of manuals on morals. I think of the poolhall proprietor in "The Last Picture Show" and of Dr. Mark Craig of "St. Elsewhere"; of Atticus Finch in *To Kill a Mockingbird* and of Trollope's wonderful old clergyman, Septimus Harding. Persis is such a person.[4]

Silas, like most entrepreneurial U.S. business people, always needed capital. Shortly after he left Vermont and came to Boston he got early, vitally necessary capital through taking a partner. The partner's name was Milton K. Rogers. Then, as soon as he could, Silas squeezed Rogers out of the company. Rogers got what his interest was worth, and that included a healthy profit; but he was forced out and the business prospered. The morals of honor would not have disapproved of the squeeze-out, then or now. But Rogers felt he had been cheated.

Persis agreed with Rogers. At her goading, Silas, after much grumbling, began lending Rogers money. The loans were really gifts (or, as Persis thought, reparations) because Silas did not expect to get the money back; the security he took was in every case worth less than the amount of the "loan."

But the security was worth something. Two parts of it are important to the story: One part was a collection of common stocks. Because of the stock, Silas began to dabble in the securities market, lost a lot, and as a result lacked the reserve capital he needed to take over the West Virginia paint mine. The other important part of Rogers's property was some undeveloped land next to a railway line in the Midwest. I will discuss the land in the next section.

When Persis was pressing Silas to be just to Rogers, she made two arguments. One was that he had cheated Rogers out of money; the other, that he forced Rogers out because making paint had become too important. The first argument was an accusation of greed; Silas, as the ethics of honor bade him to do, said there was a difference between greed and "business chance." Persis said, "You crowded him out. A man that had saved you! No, you got greedy, Silas."

Persis's other argument was that Silas was becoming an idolater: "You made paint your god, and you couldn't bear to let anybody else share in its blessings," Persis said. Persis did not say money had become a god. Money *can* become a god; Dietrichson thought that was the late nineteenth-century American business story. But money was never particularly important to the Laphams, even though Silas boasted about his wealth and tended to think he could buy good taste. Persis' accusation about money was that Silas was just ordinarily selfish.

Paint, not money, was the god; business was the *image*, and Silas wanted Rogers out of it. The issue Persis' charge raised was whether the description I attempted above, of the business as an Aristotelian practice, is wrong, and idolatry is right.[5]

The story says that Persis was being strident—probably because she wanted to be heard. Silas was not an easy person to live with; it was not always easy to get his attention. But she was mistaken; idolatry was never a serious risk for Silas Lapham. If he perceived it as a risk—particularly after Persis got his attention by saying to him that paint was his god— Silas was quick to remove the idol. When he was interviewed by the jejune Bartley Hubbard for *The Events*, Hubbard asked him if he had ever put any of his paint on his conscience. "No, sir," Silas said. "I guess you want to keep that as free from paint as you can."

What Silas liked about business, most of what made it a useful thing for him to do, was the simplicity and *clarity* of it. The normally prosaic Howells even allowed himself a symbol on the point. When the workers were driving the piles for the new house in Back Bay, Silas and Persis stopped to watch, and Silas looked at the steam-driven pile driver:

> It pleased him to hear the portable engine chuckle out a hundred thin whiffs of steam in carrying the big iron weight to the top of the framework above the pile, then seem to hesitate, and cough once or twice in pressing the weight against the detaching apparatus. There was a moment in which the weight had the effect of poising before it fell; then it dropped with a mighty whack on the iron-bound head of the pile, and drove it a foot into the earth.

"By gracious!" he would say, "there ain't anything like that in *this* world for *business*, Persis!"

As his collaboration with Tom Corey shows, Silas's business was a practice, something worthwhile to do for its own sake, among people who took it seriously. It was a form of friendship and, as such, a school for virtue.[6]

Perhaps Persis was not mistaken in thinking that Silas had, as the Laphams saw it, cheated Rogers out of some of his business profit. The ethics of honor among business gentlemen in Boston would have agreed with Silas's "business chance" position on that issue, but the problem with that resolution was that Silas did not believe it himself. But Persis' pressing the point so relentlessly, and Silas's over-reaction to it, resulted in "loans" that took capital out of the business and caused Silas to speculate in the securities market and lose even more. Persis finally decided she had pressed too hard. She decided she had made a mistake.

The fact that Persis made a mistake does not, though, have to do with Silas's business failure; failure was a circumstance. The point I want to make has to do with Persis' ability to be Silas's and their daughters' moral teacher: Persis' mistake was that she placed more importance than Silas did on the money Rogers lost when he was squeezed out, and accused Silas too much. When she came to see what she had done, she was so remorseful about it that she was unable to help Silas when he dealt with the English land buyers, when, as he saw it, he needed her most (of which more in the next section). "She came back to this, with her helpless longing, inbred in all Puritan souls, to have someone specifically suffer for the evil in the world, even if it must be herself."

That is an interesting development in the story, and it is instructive for teachers of virtue. It brings to mind Karl Barth's advice, that the person who undertakes to counsel must be prepared to be counseled. But there is a further lesson in this story about Persis disqualifying herself, for a while, as a moral teacher. In characteristic Howells fashion, it comes out of what happens next. (Character even has its uses for the ills and cures of the daily round.)

Silas did not get the advice and support he needed from Persis when he dealt with the English land buyers, but he acted virtuously anyway. Does that mean that Persis did not help him—was not his friend—did not collaborate in the good? That is what she thought: "She was so rooted in her old remorse... that she was helpless...when he had the utmost need for her insight. He had counted upon her...just spirit to stay his own in its struggle to be just...but...she was silent against him." Nonetheless, Silas came through that moral moment with character intact. He behaved as, by that time, we expected he would behave.

Silas behaved as he did because he was a virtuous person. Virtue does not operate the way moral principles do. Virtue is not in a reference book or a first-aid kit kept handy in case of moral crisis. Silas would have suffered from lack of Persis' help if he had been depending on a principle. But virtue is mundane and habitual. Silas acted as he did in the large matter of the English buyers because he had learned, from his teacher, to behave with truthfulness, justice and courage in small matters. Habit pulled him through, and that means Persis supported him even when she thought she had not.[7]

Seeing as Moral Art

Silas took the midwestern land from Rogers in partial satisfaction of part of Rogers's debt to him, then learned that the land was virtually worthless. The original attractiveness of the land as an investment had to do with the fact that it was next to a railway line; it had very little value otherwise. The local railroad company, which would have depended upon and courted whatever business an enterprise on the land might have brought to it, had sold out to a giant competitor, The Great Lacustrine & Polar Railroad.

The relative situation with the GL&P was the opposite of what it had been with the small railroad. The GL&P could, in those days, refuse to carry anything to or from Rogers's (now Silas's) land, and that meant it could render the land useless. It could buy the land for whatever price it wanted, either from Silas or from any subsequent owner.

Silas cursed Rogers. Rogers said he would find buyers for the land; Silas did not believe Rogers, but Rogers came up with two English businessmen who said they were interested in the land. Silas pondered and argued with Persis, wondering if he had to tell the English buyers about the railroad. As was usually the case, he blustered at Persis for being impractical and then concluded she was right: "[W]e might as well knock these parties down on the street, and take the money out of their pockets," he said—after the lesson.

Then Silas found out that the English buyers already knew about the GL&P, and that they were still willing to pay him a handsome price for the land. He marvelled at his good fortune, then thought about it, and then realized that Rogers and the English buyers were working together on a scheme to bilk investors in England, for whom the buyers were acting. The question then was whether Silas had to worry about the investors in England, whether he could sell the land without regard to the effect the sale might have on their investment. This was the question on which Persis was unable to speak, but on which Silas came out all right anyway.

The scene in which this is worked out is high drama. Silas has indicated to the English buyers that he is reluctant to sell (even though the sale might bring enough money to save the paint business). Rogers comes to the Lapham home and pleads with him. He has worked out a way to save Silas's conscience. He proposes that Silas sell the land back to him then Silas will not have to worry about what he does with the land. (Rogers will, of course, sell it to the English buyers.)

"It was perfectly true," Howells says. "Any lawyer would have told him the same. [Silas] could not help admiring Rogers for his ingenuity, and every selfish interest of his nature joined with many obvious duties to urge him to consent." He began to think that he was, in his scruples, standing alone—and standing alone for nothing. Persis had nothing to say.

Rogers says he would be ruined unless he could put the deal together, and that Rogers's wife (whom Silas knows to be unwell) would die of untreated illness. He tells Silas that the English investors plan to found a colony on the land; their interest, therefore, would not be affected by whether the railroad would cooperate with them or not. He points out that the GL&P has not expressed interest in the midwestern land and that the chance the railroad would control its value is remote; even if the railroad were to show an interest in the land, there would be no reason to believe it would be rapacious. He notes that the English investors are many, and wealthy; even if they lose money they would not feel the loss.

Most of those arguments were plausible, and the circumstances were powerful for accepting what was plausible. The paint business was failing; Silas had three people directly dependent on his income and many families dependent on his business; he prided himself on the fact that the "works" in Lapham had never been shut down, that the workers there had never been laid off.

When I am honest with myself, I admit that I have talked myself into doing things with less persuasion than this. If that is your experience, perhaps you will have seen what my argument is on this fourth point about virtue in business life: how important it is to see facts clearly, to know what is happening.[8]

Silas was able to handle all of Rogers's arguments, these invitations to self-deception, because he had been trained to see clearly and to tell himself the truth. Those qualities are important managerial qualities; apprentices in business are told about them and come to talk about them—frequently. My fourth argument here is mostly a matter of seeing that clear sight is as relevant to the moral life as it is to management:

"At the level of serious common sense and of ordinary nonphilosophical reflection about the nature of morals," Iris Murdoch said, "it is perfectly obvious that goodness is connected with knowledge...with a refined and honest perception of what is really the case, a patient and just discernment and exploration of what confronts one, that is the result not simply of opening one's eyes but of a certain perfectly familiar kind of moral discipline."

Murdoch describes two aspects of seeing as a moral art. First of all, it is a skill—"refined and honest perception" is the result, not of looking, but of being formed in the good habit of seeing "what is really the case." And, second, seeing as a moral art is something one learns from a teacher. When a person has learned it well—as Silas had, from his teacher, Persis—it is both ordinary and remarkable. When Silas warns Tom Corey away from investing in the paint business, he does so against his interest and against his own hearty Yankee instinct for survival. He does it even against his settled, operating, business policy that Lapham Paint will survive if it can attract capital. But there is something—I am suggesting it is a learned habit—that causes Silas to see through his policy, his interest, and his instinct, and to refuse Tom's help.

Silas suffers with Rogers's reasons for selling; Persis hears him pace the floor all through the night and is not able to say anything to him. When Rogers comes back the next morning, Silas refuses to sell. "God help my poor wife!" Rogers says. Silas watches Rogers walk away, and feels no satisfaction at all (as he might have, perhaps, if Persis had spoken up, so that he might have been able to feel her approval and to describe his refusal with a principle). "This was his reward for standing firm for right and justice to his own destruction: to feel like a thief and a murderer."

Conclusion

Most of those who tell and interpret stories about people in business in the United States seem to me to make two mistakes. The first mistake shows up in some version of the proposition that the very decision to participate in business is tragic—tragic because business is morally destructive. The second mistake says that business is esoteric; business is not destructive, but those who flourish in business are a priesthood initiated into rituals and manners that are not accessible to others.

The advantage William Dean Howells has as a teller of American business stories is that he is not interested in either the tragic or the gnostic. He stays with the ordinary. He tells in *The Rise of Silas Lapham*, and elsewhere, of plausibly ordinary, country people who come to town. He uses a relatively bucolic perspective to challenge the notions that business is tragic or esoteric. Silas and Persis Lapham are not romantics; they do not seek to find moral situations in life that pose a choice between evil and penury. And they do not know anything about "the economic order."[9]

Owen Wister said that the core of Silas's story was in Persis's focus on the way Silas treated Rogers. I am not sure that is right, and I find more complexity in her treatment of Silas on that score than Wister did. But Wister's comment is nonetheless the way to end this essay, because it says well that Howells answered theories of tragedy and priesthood with an insistence on the ordinary:[10]

> Silas obstinately justifies himself by what is called the ethics of business....Well, it didn't satisfy Mrs. Lapham. The partner was dropped at the moment when huge profits were imminent, and Silas got all of them. She...always returns to the charge.... [I]n the end, after adversity, and through it, Silas rejects a transaction which business ethics would entirely justify....This...is a good instance of that moral measure and test of human conduct which makes the foundation of all the serious writing of Howells. Conscience had not been stricken from the dictionary of his generation.[11]

Notes

1. These are not a *test* of the *validity* of the story for ethics, but are ways to draw from the story a somewhat systematic account of the ethics of virtue. Testing a story is a different project, one that rests on what I think of as the intuition we gain from a "master" story.

2. A U.S. business myth cherishes the notion that business is not a priesthood in the way the professions are, that its credentials are wit and energy and not any sort of ordination from anybody. The importance of the myth may suggest that what I am describing as the deficient view of business is today more a logical necessity for my theory than a fact. We all know "self-made men" in business, but when I was young we seemed to have known more of them. My experience and observation is that fewer people enter and advance

in business who are not inducted through graduate business school or law school or an engineering equivalent of these. If that perception is realistic, it may suggest it is a parallel to what nineteenth-century urban business gatekeepers would have defined in terms of manner, status, or membership.

3. The most thorough demonstration is in Wyatt-Brown's study of the South. Fingarette and Hauerwas are seminal sources on self-deception.

4. My son Ed reminds me also of Will Tweedy's grandfather in Olive Ann Burns's *Cold Sassy Tree*.

5. An Aristotelian practice will not be or become a god, because it is teleological: It points beyond itself. A good life will not become a god either, because a good life and idolatry are not consistent with one another: Idolatry is a matter of morals. Even the good person who does not believe in God does not put a god where God ought to be. An idolatrous life cannot, by definition, be good.

6. The theological criteria Karl Barth offered for the goodness of work in friendship reach both aspects of this argument. They are criteria which, as Barth put it, affirm our creaturely existence: (1) objectively (does justice to the objectives which have been set for it); (2) worth (does not corrupt human life; (3) humanity (regard for the work of others); (4) "reflectivity" (the "internal dimension...relation to the human soul"); and (5) limitation (limited importance)—"Work affirms human existence only because God has already affirmed human existence.")

7. Habit was important in Howell's moral theology. In *A Modern Instance*, his lawyer-character, Atherton, says, "[I]t's the implanted goodness that saves—the seed of righteousness treasured from generation to generation, and carefully watched and tended by disciplined fathers and mothers in the hearts where they have dropped it."

8. Silas would, I think, have difficulty with Professor McCoy's "federal" theory of the virtues—mostly because of issues of truthfulness, perception and self-deception. The difference between the Aristotelian account of Silas's virtues that I attempt here and a "federal" account is that the Aristotelian account points to virtue as habit, as cultural, learned, formed, acquired in a "natural," earthy way. Silas's character was, in those ways, stubborn, Yankee and Puritan. A "federal" theory of virtue would have bade him negotiate, come to terms with the moral perceptions of others, including perceptions that depend on seeing as a moral art. I think Silas would have resisted negotiation, even with a person more morally admirable than Rogers. I think he would have said that, when the going gets rough in business life, "federal" ethics looks a lot like selling out.

9. Henry Steele Commager said that Howells was at odds with "the economic order," that he did not like it and, as a result, did not understand it. Howells's strength as a business storyteller was the personal: "He never really

understood the order which he hated as he understood the order which he loved; perhaps it was because he was so poor at hate and so generous in love." Another way to make that point would be to say that Silas liked doing business, and he was proud of his paint, but he did not understand "the economic order" either.

10. "The ethics of business" is the ethic of the priesthood, what I have called here an ethic of honor.

11. I am grateful for the assistance of Michael Goldberg, Patricia O'Hara, Kathleen Sullivan, and Edward, Joseph and Nancy Shaffer.

Bibliography

Aristotle, *Nichomachean Ethics*, trans. Martin Ostwald (Indianapolis: Bobbs-Merrill, 1962).

Barth, Karl, *Church Dogmatics*, (Edinburgh: T. and T. Clark, 1961) (on work), vol. III/4, pp. 516-534.

Barth, Karl, *The Humanity of God*, (Atlanta: John Knox Press, 1960) (on counseling), pp. 86-87.

Cady, Edwin H., and Frazier, David L., eds., *The War of the Critics over William Dean Howells* (Evanston: Row, Peterson and Company, 1962).

Colohan, Rev. John Francis, M.M., "The Portrayal of the Moral World in the Novels of William Dean Howells," doctoral dissertation in the Department of English, University of Notre Dame, June 1951.

Cook, Don L., ed., *William Dean Howells, The Rise of Silas Lapham: An Authoritative Text, Composition and Backgrounds, Contemporary Responses [and] Criticism* (New York: Norton, 1982).

Commager, Henry Steel, "The Return to Howells," *The Spectator*, May 28, 1948, vol. 180, p. 642; in Cady and Frazier, pp. 191, 193.

Dietrichson, Jan, *The Image of Money in the American Novel of the Gilded Age* (New York: Humanities Press, 1969).

Fingarette, Herbert, *Self-Deception* (Atlantic Highlands, NJ: Humanities Press, 1969).

Firkins, Oscar W., *William Dean Howells: A Study* (Cambridge, MA: Harvard University Press, 1924).

Goldberg, Michael, *Jews and Christians: Getting Our Stories Straight (The Exodus and the Passion-Resurrection)* (Nashville: Abingdon, 1985).

Goldberg, Michael, *Theology and Narrative: A Critical Introduction* (Nashville: Abingdon, 1982).

Halfmann, Ulrich, *Interviews with William Dean Howells* (Arlington, TX: University of Texas, 1973).

Hauerwas, Stanley, *Truthfulness and Tragedy* (Notre Dame, IN: University of Notre Dame Press, 1977).

Howells, William Dean (on tragedy); see Halfmann.

MacIntyre, Alasdair, *After Virtue*, 2nd ed. (Notre Dame, IN: University of Notre Dame Press, 1984).

Mason, Philip, *The English Gentleman: The Rise and Fall of an Ideal* (1982) (includes material from John Henry Newman).

Miller, Arthur, *All My Sons* (New York: Dramatists Play Service, Inc., 1974).

Murdoch, Iris, *The Sovereignty of Good* (1970) (London: Ark ed., 1985).

Newman, John Henry; see Mason.

Scudder, H.E., "The Rise of Silas Lapham," *Atlantic Monthly*, October 1885, vol. 56, p. 554; and "Mr. Howells's Literary Creed," *Atlantic Monthly*, October 1891, vol. 68, p. 566; in Cady and Frazier, pp. 26, 61.

Shaffer, Thomas L., *Faith and the Professions* (Provo, UT: Brigham Young University, 1987).

Shaffer, Thomas L., *On Being a Christian and a Lawyer* (Provo, UT: Brigham Young University Press, 1980).

Shaffer, Thomas L., *American Legal Ethics* (New York: Matthew Bender, 1985).

Siker, L. van Wensveen, "An Unlikely Dialogue: Barth and Business Ethicists on Human Work," in D.M. Yeager, ed., *The Annual of the Society of Christian Ethics*, 131-145 (Washington, D.C.: Georgetown University Press, 1989).

Wister, Owen, "William Dean Howells," *Atlantic Monthly*, December 1937, vol. 160, p. 704; in Cady and Frazier, pp. 178, 181-182.

Wyatt-Brown, Bertram, *Southern Honor: Ethics and Behavior in the Old South* (New York: Oxford University Press, 1982).

Contributors

Michael G. Bowen is an assistant professor of management at the University of Notre Dame. He has published in *Academy of Management Review, Principles and Applications of Information Science for Library Professionals* and *World's Fair.*

C. Samuel Calian is president of the Pittsburgh Theological Seminary and founding director of the Center for Ethics and Social Policy, Berkeley, and the Trinity Center for Ethics and Corporate Policy, New York. He is the author of *The Significance of Eschatology in the Thoughts of Nicolas Berdyaev; Berdyaev's Philosophy of Hope; Icon and Pulpit; Grace, Guts and Goods; The Gospel According to the Wall Street Journal; Today's Pastor in Tomorrow's World; For All Your Seasons: Biblical Direction Through Life's Passages;* and *Where Is the Passion for Excellence in the Church?*

Krishna S. Dhir is a professor and the director of the School of Business Administration at the Pennsylvania State University in Harrisburg. He has published in *International Journal of Hospitality Management, Perspectives in Hydrobiology, Academic Chairpersons: In Search of Academic Quality, Decision Line, Healthcare Human Resource Forum, Handbook of Behavioral Economics, Global Issues of Information Technology Management* and *Telematics India.*

Michael Goldberg of McKinsey & Company, Inc., in Atlanta, Georgia, is the author of *Theology and Narrative* and *Jews and Christians, Getting Our Stories Straight,* and editor of *A Consultation on Professionalism and the Law,* and *The Practice of Law: Is There Anything More to It Than Making Money?*

John W. Houck is a professor of management and co-director of the Notre Dame Center for Ethics and Religious Values in Business at the University of Notre Dame. He is the author of *Academic Freedom and the Catholic University, Outdoor Advertising: History and Regulation* and *A Matter of*

Dignity: Inquiries into the Humanization of Work, and co-author of *Full Value: Cases in Christian Business Ethics*. He is co-editor of *The Judeo-Christian Vision and the Modern Corporation, Co-Creation and Capitalism: John Paul II's Laborem Exercens, Catholic Social Teaching and the U.S. Economy: Working Papers for a Bishops' Pastoral, The Common Good and U.S. Capitalism, Ethics and the Investment Industry* and *The Making of an Economic Vision*.

Dennis P. McCann is a professor of religious studies and co-director of the Center for the Study of Values at DePaul University. He is the author of *Christian Realism and Liberation Theology* and *New Experiment in Democracy: The Challenge for American Catholicism*, and co-author of *Polity and Praxis: A Program for American Practical Theology*. He is co-editor of *On Moral Business: Religious and Theological Perspectives on Business, Ethics, and Society*.

Charles S. McCoy is the Robert Gordon Sprout professor of theological ethics at the Pacific School of Religion. He is the author of *The Meaning of Theological Reflection, The Covenant Theology of Johannes Cocceius, The Responsible Campus: Toward a New Identity for the Church-Related College, Ethics in the Corporate Policy Process: An Introduction, The Covenant in America: Renewing Our Expectations, When Gods Change: Hope for Theology, History, Humanity, and Federalism in the Theology and Ethics of Johannes Cocceius, Götter Ändern sich: Hoffnung für die Theologie, Management of Values: The Ethical Difference in Corporate Policy and Performance*, and *Managing Values: A Practical Guide for Executives* (in progress).

Patrick E. Murphy is a professor and chairman of the department of marketing at the University of Notre Dame. He has published articles on business and marketing ethics in the *Journal of Marketing, Journal of Macromarketing, Journal of Business Ethics, Advances in Marketing and Public Policy* and *Sloan Management Review*. He has also published *Marketing Ethics: Guidelines for Managers* and *The Higher Road: A Path to Ethical Marketing Decisions*.

F. Clark Power is an associate professor of education and developmental psychology at the University of Notre Dame. He is the principal author of

Lawrence Kohlberg's Approach to Moral Education and co-author of *The Measurement of Moral Judgment*. He is co-editor of *Self, Ego, and Identity: Integrative Approaches* and *The Challenge of Pluralism: Education, Politics, and Values*.

Thomas L. Shaffer is the Robert and Marion Short professor of law at the University of Notre Dame Law School. He is the author of *The Planning and Drafting of Wills and Trusts, Legal Interviewing and Counseling in a Nutshell, On Being a Christian and a Lawyer: Law for the Innocent* and *Faith and the Professions*, and co-author of *Legal Interviewing and Counseling Cases* and *American Lawyers and Their Communities: Ethics in the Legal Profession*.

Oliver F. Williams, C.S.C., is an associate provost and co-director of the Notre Dame Center for Ethics and Religious Values in Business at the University of Notre Dame. He is the author of *The Apartheid Crisis: How We Can Do Justice in a Land of Violence* and co-author of *Full Value: Cases in Christian Business Ethics*. He is co-editor of *The Judeo-Christian Vision and the Modern Corporation, Co-Creation and Capitalism: John Paul II's Laborem Exercens, Catholic Social Teaching and the U.S. Economy: Working Papers for a Bishops' Pastoral, The Common Good and U.S. Capitalism, Ethics and the Investment Industry* and *The Making of an Economic Vision*.